D1229666

lightenUP

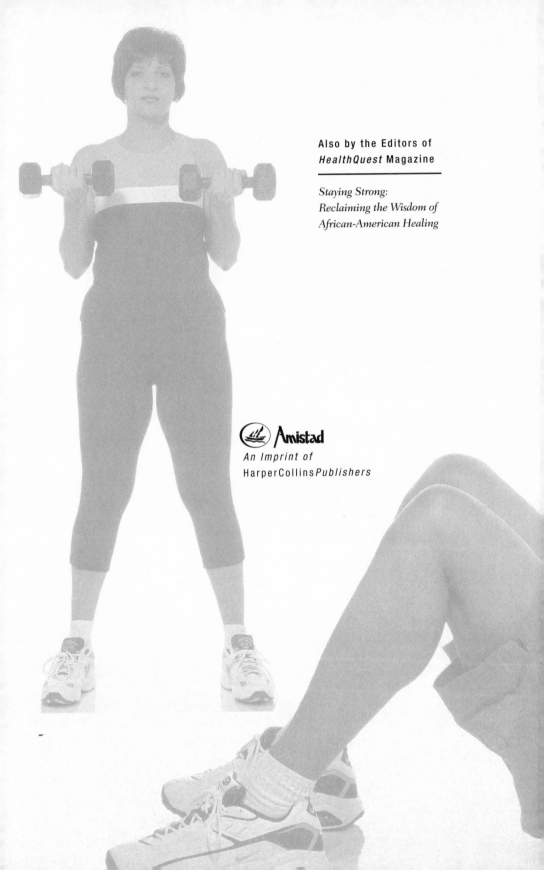

Also by the Editors of
HealthQuest **Magazine**

Staying Strong:
Reclaiming the Wisdom of
African-American Healing

Amistad
An Imprint of
HarperCollins*Publishers*

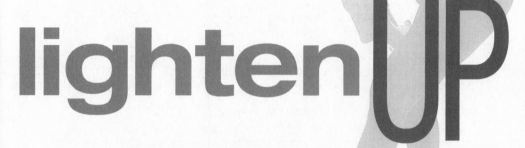

lightenUP

The *HealthQuest* 30-Day Weight-Loss Program

The Editors of *HealthQuest* Magazine
with Therman E. Evans, M.D.

Photography by Welton Doby III

This book is written as a source of information only. The information contained in this book should by no means be considered a substitute for the advice of a qualified medical professional, who should always be consulted before beginning any new diet, exercise, or other health program. All efforts have been made to ensure the accuracy of the information contained in this book as of the date published. The author and the publisher expressly disclaim responsibility for any adverse effects arising from the use or application of the information contained herein.

LIGHTEN UP. Copyright © 2001 by LEVAS, Inc. Recipes by Goulda Downer, Ph.D., R.D., C.N.S., Metroplex Health and Nutrition Services, Inc., Washington, D.C.

All rights reserved. Printed in the United States of America. No part of this book may be used or reproduced in any manner whatsoever without written permission except in the case of brief quotations embodied in critical articles and reviews. For information, address HarperCollins Publishers Inc., 10 East 53rd Street, New York, NY 10022.

HarperCollins books may be purchased for educational, business, or sales promotional use. For information, please write: Special Markets Department, HarperCollins Publishers Inc., 10 East 53rd Street, New York, NY 10022.

FIRST EDITION

DESIGNED BY DEBORAH KERNER

PHOTOGRAPHY BY WELTON DOBY III

Printed on acid-free paper

Library of Congress Cataloging-in-Publication Data

Lighten Up: the HealthQuest 30-day weight-loss program /
by the editors of HealthQuest magazine
with Therman E. Evans, M.D.
p.   m.
Includes index.
ISBN 0-380-97561-0
1. Weight loss.   2. African Americans—Health and hygiene.
I. Evans, Therman E.   II. HealthQuest.

RM222.2.L477 2001

613.7'089'96073—dc21   2001022628

01 02 03 04 05 / RRD / 10 9 8 7 6 5 4 3 2 1

Contents

Foreword

As a physician, I see many people with health and medical challenges, the majority of whom are African-American. Black people have higher mortality rates from deaths in all of the major disease areas—heart disease, cancer, diabetes, and HIV/AIDS, as well as homicide and infant deaths—than other racial and ethnic groups. We become ill and die so disproportionately that I find it painful to witness.

The irony is that these excessive rates of death and disease can be alleviated—even prevented—by positive lifestyle changes, such as losing weight, engaging in a regular exercise routine, managing stress, reducing sugar and salt consumption, and maintaining a healthy diet that includes eating more fruits and vegetables.

Of course, all of these lifestyle adjustments require that people adopt new behaviors. People who are willing to change can dramatically improve their health. However, we humans are creatures of habit; we just *don't* like to change, even when it means things will be better. That's why the *need* for change does not necessarily *bring* change. Most people require some kind of catalyst.

So the question becomes, What does it take for a person to make changes beneficial to his or her health? Some people change once exposed to new information, but these individuals seem to be few and far between. More often, people seem to need a far more dramatic stimulus—the illness or death of a loved one, for instance, or a personal illness or tragedy. We hope to convince you to change before any health crisis strikes you or someone you love. But no matter how severe a catalyst you require, one thing is certain: Positive lifestyle behavior changes are essential to achieving good health and well-being.

Eating a proper diet and maintaining a healthy weight are both essential to good health. Heart disease, cancer, and diabetes are all strongly influenced by overeating and poor diet. Eating too much food, as well as eating foods that are high in fat and sugar, also contributes to one of the most common medical risk factors—obesity.

Obesity is epidemic in America. It is the most common form of malnutrition found in our society. According to the Mayo Clinic, one in four Americans is considered obese, and 55 percent of Americans over age twenty (one out of every two) are considered overweight or obese. Research indicates that obesity has become so epidemic in this country that there are probably as many overweight people here as there are underfed people on the entire planet.

Many people feel that carrying excess weight is more of a social than a medical problem. Unfortunately, they are sadly mistaken. Obesity has tremendous negative health implications. In 1991 the *Journal of the American Medical Association* reported that about three hundred thousand Americans die from obesity-related illnesses each year—illnesses like high blood pressure, diabetes, coronary heart disease, stroke, gall bladder disease, and certain cancers. Obesity can also cause less dramatic problems that, nevertheless, reduce one's quality of life: breathing problems, low-back pain, swelling of the feet and ankles, arthritis in joints such as the hips and the knees. Because African-Americans have such high levels of obesity, we're disproportionately affected by these conditions, too.

Taking weight off and keeping it off will significantly reduce your risk factors for these health problems by helping to lower your blood pressure, blood cholesterol, blood sugar, and the stress and strain on the joints of the hip and lower extremities.

By following the advice in this book, you will be able to do just that. There is no extreme, "miracle," or fad diet presented here. Instead, you'll find a sound, reasonable, commonsensical holistic approach to weight loss and weight management.

The *HealthQuest* 30-Day Weight-Loss Program begins right where you are and gradually transports you to lifestyle changes that will result in the health and well-being you desire. It is easy to implement because it builds upon your current eating and exercising habits. As you adjust your lifestyle to incorporate the program's recommendations, you will be amazed and inspired by the results. Not only will you improve your general health, you'll create a better-functioning, and better-looking, body.

Determine to begin today.

Yours in good health,

THERMAN E. EVANS, M.D.

Preface

I never had a weight problem growing up. I was an athletic child and an active teenager. Even through college, when I exercised less frequently, I was never weight obsessed. So when I got pregnant at age thirty with my first child, I wasn't particularly concerned that over the course of nine months my 5'3" frame began to steadily expand. I shrugged it off to the fact that I was surely having a "big baby" and carrying excess water weight. (The baby ended up being only 6 pounds, 15 ounces.)

As a self-admitted sweet freak, I looked at pregnancy as the rare time in a woman's life when she could indulge in all her food obsessions. For me, it was dessert after every meal. Hey, I was eating for two. By week forty, I had gained a whopping fifty pounds. Thirty of it came off immediately. But losing that other twenty was a two-year journey of re-educating my mind and body. Of course, as soon as I reached my goal weight I got pregnant with my second child. This time around I gained only forty pounds.

And here I am today, still on the journey. What I understand now is that weight management is not a temporary process. We have to be ever vigilant and always mindful of what, when, and how much we eat—and, often, why. And we have to incorporate exercise into our lives.

It's not easy fitting it all in. But it has to be a priority. We must claim time for caring for our own bodies, minds, and spirits. Only then can we adequately care for our loved ones.

We offer *Lighten Up* as a guide to successful, long-term, healthy weight loss. It is borne out of our personal experiences and the tremendous expertise that exists in the African-American health and nutrition arena. With more than 50 percent of Black women fighting obesity in one way, shape, or form, we had to write this book at this moment in time. It is part of *HealthQuest* magazine's mission: to uplift, encourage, and inspire our community of readers to take charge of their well-being.

I want to acknowledge the many contributors who poured their time and talent into the pages of this book. First, I would like to thank Hilary Beard, who as *HealthQuest*'s managing editor used her writing and editing skills to ensure that *Lighten Up* was thorough, accurate, and, above all, user-friendly for our many readers. Thanks to Kirk Johnson and Tamara Jeffries for their writing and editing expertise that give this book a fun, energetic voice that we hope inspires our readers to make a change; Constance Brown-Riggs, our incredibly knowledgeable and resourceful registered dietitian who analyzed and developed the nutritional components of the *HealthQuest* weight-loss plan; Dr. Goulda Downer, a phenomenal nutritionist and talented chef who developed the delicious recipes showcased in this book; Jeanne Humphrey, who provided essential technical assistance and administrative support; Manie Baron and John Jusino, our editors at HarperCollins, who shepherded this book through the intricate publishing maze; Therman Evans, M.D., who made sure we approached this book holistically and that we were on point medically; the *HealthQuest* staff for being dedicated to the magazine's overall mission; and my family for allowing me to continue to step out on faith and create new works.

We offer this book as a tool for personal enhancement and growth. Use it wisely and well.

SARA LOMAX REESE
Publisher, *HealthQuest* Magazine

Introduction

Toward a New Program: Understanding Your Ancestral Diet and Your Health

First, let's get one thing straight: This is not your ordinary diet. This is a weight-loss program that deals with more than just food; the *HealthQuest* 30-Day Weight-Loss Program will teach you how to lose weight and how to keep it off by mobilizing your mind, body, and spirit to make healthy lifestyle changes that you can implement now and maintain forever.

If you've ever wanted to lose more than a few pounds, you've probably tried most diets on the planet: The fad diets that fail. (Remember the Grapefruit Diet? And all that cabbage soup?) The ones based on unsubstantiated claims. ("The Potato Chip Diet: Eat all you want and never gain a pound!"). The expensive "you'll lose only if you eat the foods we sell" diets. ("All you have to do is come in and stock up for the week.") And you may have experienced the broken promises ("Burn fifty pounds of fat your first month!") and the Re-run Routine (when your diet goes belly-up and you watch the weight you lost come creeping right back).

Usually when diets fail, we're quick to blame ourselves instead of the diet. And so we move on to the next fad diet, always hoping, always dreaming—and always disappointed, oftentimes in ourselves.

At *HealthQuest: Total Wellness for Body, Mind and Spirit,* we know the frustration that goes hand in hand with dieting—and we promise not to put you through that unnecessary pain and suffering. We're going to teach you how to change your lifestyle in a way that helps you lose weight and keep it off! And we're going to teach you how to do so in manageable, thirty-day increments that you can repeat for as long as you want to lose weight.

Sure, you'll have to take a close look at your food choices and make some changes. But we'll show you how to evaluate your current eating habits and plan healthier menus, and we'll even give you some scrumptious, low-fat, low-calorie recipes to use, all with the flavors and ingredients we adore.

You'll also have to get off the couch and get some exercise—but relax. You won't have to buy a lot of fancy equipment or join some exclusive fitness club. During your *HealthQuest* 30-Day Weight-Loss Program, we'll show you how to make fitness a fun and affordable part of losing weight.

But perhaps most important, you'll begin to get yourself in the right frame of mind to keep the weight off. That means using the mental capacity you were born with and the spiritual strength that's fortified Americans of African descent for many generations to inspire and support the changes you're making for your body. Because when it's body, mind, *and* spirit against fat—fat loses every time.

Eating with the Enemy

Aaah, fat—the bacon grease we use to scramble our eggs, the vegetable oil that sizzles our fries, the full-fat Cheddar cheese that drips from Mama's macaroni. The same fat that jiggles around our middles, rides side-saddle on our thighs and keeps on flapping after we've waved our loved ones good-bye.

As convenient as it is to order fast-food for take-out, as proud as you may be of your ability to replicate Big Mama's Down-Home Double-Butter Pound Cake, as protective as you are of the secret you possess to grilling perfect ribs, if you're reading this book, you've probably already acknowledged that some of your eating habits have come with a price tag. If you're lucky, the price is only excess weight; if you're not so lucky, that weight may have put your health at risk.

Either way, you're not alone. America is experiencing a weight-gain epidemic. According to the Centers for Disease Control and Prevention (CDC), between 1960 and 1999 (the most recent year for which government data is available), the percentage of Americans considered obese increased from 13 to 26 percent. And the rate at which we're gaining weight has accelerated rapidly in recent years.

In 1987 there was no state in the country in which 15 percent of the population was considered obese—roughly 30 pounds overweight, or a Body Mass Index (BMI) greater than or equal to 30 (more on BMI later). By 1991 this had increased to six states. And by 1998, this weight gain had exploded to forty-five states. Also in 1998, twelve states reported to the federal government that between 33 and 51 percent of their populations engaged in no leisure-time physical activity—an all-time low.

And while this epidemic of weight gain is reflected across every race and socioeconomic group, sisters are putting on more weight than anyone else, including African-American men. The CDC's National Health and Nutrition Examination Survey completed in 1992 found that 49 percent of Black women were overweight (BMI greater than or equal to 25) versus 32 percent of White women. And while high, the percentage of Black men who were overweight (31 percent) was consistent with the percentage of both White men (32 percent) and White women (32 percent).

Another CDC study, published in 1997, showed that 64.5 percent of Black women were overweight and that the rate had increased by 9 percent in just ten years. (Prior to that, government statistics showed that the percentage of sisters who were overweight had hovered consistently in the low 40 percent range since 1960.) The same study showed that this phenomenon of weight gain also affected Black men. In the 1980s, the percentage of Black men who were overweight increased from the low 20 percent range, where it had held steady since the mid-'60s, to 34 percent in the mid-'90s. The percentage of Black men who are overweight is consistent with the overall population, but it, too, is increasing rapidly. Excess fat is plaguing America, but it is literally *killing* the African-American community—and the enemy is right at the end of our fork.

Now, at *HealthQuest*, we want to encourage and empower you to take charge of your health. And we don't want to scare you half to death or to bury you in statistics. But we love our people too much to spare you the truth. So we're gonna give you the skinny on the dangers of fat and make you aware of the unique set of circumstances that have put us in this position. Then we're going to show you how to do something about it.

What's at Stake

As we move into the twenty-first century, "Black Americans have a life expectancy of seventy-two [years], compared to the national average of seventy-seven," says Surgeon General David Satcher, M.D., Ph.D. Not only do we live shorter lives, the quality of our lives is often compromised because we are stricken disproportionately with disease, become sick at a younger age, and experience more debilitating symptoms than our White peers.

It probably won't surprise you to know that heart disease, cancer, and stroke, the top three causes of death in the United States, hit African-Americans hardest. According to the American Heart Association (AHA), Black men and women are 46 percent and 67 percent more likely to die of heart disease and stroke, respectively, than our White peers of the same age. Approximately 35 percent of the African-American population suffers from hypertension, a major risk factor for stroke, compared to 24 percent of the general United States population, according to a study published in 1999 in the *Journal of the National Medical Association*.

We also suffer disproportionately from cancer. According to the American Cancer Society, while the death rate for cancer declined significantly across all racial groups between 1990 through 1995, African-Americans still die from cancer more often than any other Americans. Lung cancer is the leading cause of cancer deaths among Black Americans. Black women die of breast cancer more often than White women, even though they get the disease less frequently. Black men and women die from colon and rectal cancer more often than any other American racial or ethnic group. And African-American men have the highest rate of prostate cancer *in the entire world*.

To make matters worse, we're also more likely to suffer and die from diabetes, the nation's seventh-leading cause of death. According to the National Diabetes Education Program, African-Americans are 27 percent more likely to die from diabetes than White Americans. By the time we turn fifty, at least 28 percent of Black women and 19 percent of Black men have the disease. (And we're starting to get it younger; diabetes incidence among children is growing at a rapid rate.) We're also more likely to experience traumatic diabetes-related health problems, such as arteriosclerosis, kidney failure, the loss of eyesight, or amputated limbs.

We don't want to be gruesome, but let's consider for a moment what all this means; let's make all those statistics plain. The commonly held image of a heart attack victim—an older White man keeling over at the office—is far from what's happening in the real world. Sisters are suffering strokes after Bible study and brothers are having heart attacks on their way home from work. We're losing our lungs, breasts, and reproductive organs at rates far higher than everyone else. And we're more likely to end up on dialysis machines, waiting for a transplant, or with amputated toes and feet. This is not how we envisioned living out our older years—and it's certainly not what we thought we would experience in middle age.

Checking Our Choices

W hy are Black folks at risk for such debilitating diseases and dispro-portionately devastating consequences? Well, sometimes things we can't control, like our environment and genetics, play a critical role. But the risk of these uncontrollable factors can be heightened or triggered—or not—by our lifestyle choices, including what we eat and how much we exercise.

On that note, here's the good news: *Almost all of these diseases—and many others—are preventable with lifestyle changes.*

Study after study shows that eating a healthy diet (one that's high in fiber, and low in fat, cholesterol, and sodium), losing excess weight, and engaging in a regular program of moderately strenuous exercise reduces your risk of devel-oping heart disease, stroke, a variety of cancers, and diabetes. According to the American Heart Association, losing as little as ten to twenty pounds can make a big difference. And exercising at a moderate to vigorous rate for as little as thirty minutes a day most days of the week (at least five) can reduce your risk of heart disease. The American Cancer Society echoes these sug-gestions, claiming that a high-fat diet contributes to about 35 percent of can-cer deaths, including cancers of the colon and rectum, prostate, and endometrium, and that regular physical activity can reduce your risk of colon and breast cancer. Several studies also suggest that smokers who eat a healthy diet (especially vegetarians who smoke) are less likely to develop lung cancer than those who consume a lot of animal protein and few fruits and vegetables.

Part of our problem is prosperity. More Americans these days can afford effort-saving (read: calorie-saving) devices. We can purchase the technology that encourages us to play ball on the computer rather than on the court. We can eat out more; we can buy more groceries. That's at least part of the reason the rates of obesity sky-rocketed almost 60 percent, from 12 percent of the population in 1991 to 19 percent by 1999.

Now the medical definition of obesity is not always the same as what the rest of us might commonly call being "fat." And even then, there are a couple of medical definitions. The federal government defines obesity as a Body Mass Index (BMI) of 30, the equivalent of being about thirty pounds overweight. (We'll teach you how to calculate your BMI in chapter 8.)

Another medical definition for obesity states that a person weighs at least 20 percent more than the "norm" for their height and bone structure (more on "norms" shortly). If you weigh 20 percent more, you're considered slightly obese; 40 percent more and you're moderately obese; at 50 percent more, you're considered morbidly obese; and at 100 pounds above the weight you should be, you're considered hyperobese. While we can—and momentarily, will—argue that norms are in the eye of the beholder, these categories are significant because they reflect the risk that excess weight poses to your health. Whether or not we agree with the majority's standard of beauty, we don't want to be so hardheaded that we jeopardize our lives.

Obesity is on the rise, among people of color especially, and Black folks are leading the pack. Centers for Disease Control (CDC) researchers have found that weight gain is most prevalent among Black women between the ages of twenty-five and thirty-four, but at every age, African-American women are significantly more likely to be obese than any other group. By the time sisters reach middle age, more than 60 percent will be obese. While 40 percent of Black men are obese by the time they reach their late thirties. That's a little better than for sisters, but still higher than average. Thirty-three percent of the U.S. population is considered obese, and Black men and women are the most obese of all major ethnic groups in the nation.

Being overweight is a prime health hazard for people who want to live long, healthy lives. In fact, it's a tragedy waiting to happen. All told, more deaths are associated with obesity than with smoking.

Obesity causes stress on other systems of the body, which causes them to become overworked, worn down, or otherwise nonfunctional. For example, excess weight taxes your cardiovascular system and can cause cholesterol levels to increase, which can lead to heart disease and hypertension. Hypertension, in turn, can cause kidney failure, stroke, or heart attack.

Excess weight can make the cells in your body insulin-resistant—unable to absorb sugar from your bloodstream—which can lead to diabetes. Obesity can make it harder for women to get pregnant and can cause complications during a cesarean section or any other kind of surgery, according to researchers at the Weight and Obesity Program at the University of

Pennsylvania. And it is linked to osteoarthritis since the joints get more wear and tear from carrying around a heavier load.

A lot of this information is not new. Still, many of us find it difficult to change. Now there are good reasons why change can be challenging—we work stressful jobs, our kids keep us busy, and there's never enough time at the end of the day. And it's not just Black folks who are getting larger; we're just the most extreme example of what is clearly an American phenomenon. According to the CDC, between 1998 and 1999, obesity in the United States rose by 6 percent, with White Americans exhibiting the greatest increase. As our society becomes more fast-paced and convenience-oriented, Americans of all stripes are replacing home-cooked meals made with fresh ingredients with fast-food, take-out, and convenience foods. These meals are often high in calories, fat, cholesterol, and sodium, all of which can be detrimental to our health. We're driving more instead of walking, we're watching TV and using computers, our jobs are more sedentary, and we're getting less physical exercise—unless we can include the workout our fingers get operating the remote control. All Americans are taking more fat and calories into their bodies and are not moving around enough to work them off.

But there are some aspects of this weight-gain epidemic that are uniquely African-American. For instance, in addition to the fast- and convenience foods that all Americans have come to rely on, we have a preference for a unique combination of ingredients and flavors known as soul food—the rich cultural legacy of our forebears—which, in addition to being delicious, is usually high in fat, cholesterol, and sodium. Even Black folks of Caribbean and African descent tend to cook with high-fat ingredients like palm oil and coconut oil. Don't expect us to eat some bland diet of boiled broccoli just because it's good for us; we expect our food to tantalize our taste buds and nourish our souls. Moreover, soul food forms the centerpiece of many of our family traditions and cultural celebrations. When we get together, it's often around food. We cling to soul food jealously, and if we're gonna consider eating something else, it had better contain the foods and flavors we love.

Black folks are also less likely to believe that there is a cause-and-effect relationship between our diet and our health, according to a study conducted by the Morehouse College of Medicine and New America Wellness. African-Americans of all ages are less active than Whites, according to data from the CDC's 1998 Behavioral Risk Factor Surveillance System. In that survey, more than one-third of African-American adults reported engaging in no leisure-time physical activity, with Black women more likely to be inactive than men. And American Heart Association studies show that after a long day of hard work, Black folks believe that downtime for rest is more important than engaging in exercise. So when we get a free moment, our tendency is to cop a squat rather than jump to the gym.

But with the devastating health catastrophe that we're facing, it is time for Black Americans of all backgrounds—and especially sisters—to begin to think about the reasons we do the things we do. Why it is, for instance, that Black folks all over the country throw down on many of the same favorite dishes—ham hocks and hog maws, collards and candied yams, macaroni and cheese and black-eyed peas? And even when confronted with the knowledge that some of these foods can be bad for our health when eaten frequently and traditionally prepared, why are many of us so resistant to change?

The foods and flavors we know as "soul food" have a longstanding history among Black folks in America—a history that helps explain why we find some foods so irresistible and that empowers us to figure out how to enjoy the flavors we love without sacrificing our health.

Where did soul food come from? And how does it differ from what our African ancestors ate? These are important questions for us to consider.

In the Beginning . . .

We may associate what we know as soul food with satisfying, soul-warming, down-home goodness. But soul food is really a culinary adaptation that allowed enslaved Africans to cling to life in a new land in which food was scarce, but violence and oppression hung abundantly from trees.

Prior to their arrival in the Americas, all people of African descent had a food history based on life in stable families, healthy communities, and a more hospitable environment. For thousands of years, our African ancestors used the earth's bounty to craft simple, nourishing meals. The food supply wasn't always guaranteed: Sometimes harvests were plentiful; sometimes they were dismal. But by and large, the typical African diet was substantial enough to sustain generations. Our bodies adapted to survive feast and famine. And if modern epidemiological evidence provides a window into the past, these traditional foods allowed Africans to enjoy impressively low rates of the chronic diseases that plague African-Americans today.

Depending on where in Africa was their ancestral homeland, our ancestors might have found a variety of different foods and flavors on their table—foods that were influenced by any of the more than eight hundred ethnic groups of Africa south of the Sahara Desert, including Arabs, Asians, Berbers, or, less likely, Europeans. But no matter where on the continent they lived, a typical diet included a low-fat, mostly vegetarian mix of leafy green vegetables, root vegetables (such as yams), beans, fruits, a variety of grains, brown breads, occasional dairy products, and small amounts of animal protein, like fish or poultry.

According to food historian Jessica B. Harris, in West Africa, the ancestral home of most Black Americans, people commonly ate turnips, cabbage, and a variety of greens; various pumpkins, calabashes, and gourds; okra, corn, and tomatoes; numerous beans and peas, including black-eyed peas, chickpeas, and lentils; many grains, like rice, millet, couscous; and porridges. Common fruits included mangos, dates, melons (including watermelon), tamarind, oranges, and lemons. And salt, a variety of peppers, ginger, onions, and garlic were usually used for seasoning. Chicken was the most frequent source of animal protein; fish was eaten along the coast and in river areas; and lamb and other red meats were used sparingly for seasoning. Most red meats were used as ingredients in a wide variety of stews, but the meat itself was not central to the meal, unless it was part of a huge feast. Food was boiled, roasted, or baked—rarely fried. Our African ancestors ate good food thoughtfully gathered and nutritiously prepared. How easy to see that many of the foods we prefer today are indigenous to our ancestral homeland.

Soul Survivor

Slavery almost destroyed Africans' culinary connection to the Motherland. A few fortunate slaves were allowed to maintain gardens for themselves or to hunt and fish during their brief breaks from fieldwork. The vegetables, meat, and fish collected this way allowed some to continue, as best as they could, their African culinary traditions in the New World. But most barely got by on slave owners' meager rations consisting primarily of cornmeal and molasses or by eating the stuff White folks threw away. Still, many captives were able to hold on to some aspects of their food heritage. Whenever possible, the captives combined the food traditions of their native lands with new practices spawned by their will to survive. *In this way, they created new food traditions.*

"When their masters ate turnips, slaves had the tough, bitter turnip greens," explains Tanya Y. Wright in the *New York Times Magazine*. "When slave owners dined on ham, bacon, and sausage—giving rise to the phrase 'high on the hog'—slaves were given the less desirable and, in some cases, fattier parts of the pig, like the shoulder ('ham hock'), feet ('trotters'), snout ('snoot'), neck, backbone, stomach, and intestines." Thus the African-American taste for pork and some of the more peculiar parts of the pig.

Black folks also developed our taste for salt during slavery times. "We salted our food to keep it from spoiling," says Goulda Downer, Ph.D., R.D., a nutritionist and dietitian in Washington, D.C. "And when it did spoil, we put more salt and spices on it to cover it up," she says. No wonder we still have a taste for salty foods today.

The desire to survive also dictated that the slaves' primary methods of cooking had to change. Rather than roasting, baking, or boiling ingredients, slaves usually were forced to fry their foods over a fireplace in a single pot. Frying was a quick and efficient cooking method. Fat was readily available from pork trimmings and provided ample calories and a feeling of fullness that lasted well into the day. Slaves were able to eat this way without the health consequences we experience today because fieldwork was so physically demanding that they worked off the fat.

So this was the origin of soul food. It's important that we all understand: The food we are so attached to—the soul food that we cling to like cornbread clings to our ribs—was not the food of our free ancestors, but a survival diet adopted by a people desperate and enslaved.

"Soul food is survival food," culinary historian Jessica Harris told Tanya Wright. "Slaves made the best of a bad lot."

The Emancipation Proclamation did little to break traditions forged during these years of hardship. Even after the end of slavery, African-Americans cooked and ate much as they did when enslaved. That meant that if you were poor—and if you were Black—you might scrape by on subsistence meals. In 1897 the U.S. Department of Agriculture (USDA) dispatched scientists to Tuskegee, Alabama, to study the dietary habits of rural Black farmers. "The food consisted almost exclusively of fat pork, corn meal, and molasses," the researchers reported. Not exactly five-star cuisine—or the right foods to nourish hard-working bodies. Still, folks did the best they could. And in parts of the country where climate and available land allowed, we brought an ample array of fresh, nutritious foods to the table.

In an interview with *HealthQuest* magazine, Lauren Swann, M.S., R.D., a Pennsylvania-based nutritional consultant, says a key difference between African-Americans' diets then and now is our lack of connectedness to the land.

"During the early part of the century, we weren't as reliant upon processed and refined foods as we are now," she says. "Sharecroppers ate off the land and even Black folks who traveled to the cities still kept gardens to grow fresh fruits and vegetables."

In fact, says Swann, meat didn't dominate African-Americans' meals until a few decades ago. "My grandmother used to go to the butcher and ask for bones for the dog. These bones would have chunks of meat still on them, and she would use them to make soup—which is not the same as sitting down to a meal of smothered pork chops every night."

Carolyn Coker-Ross, M.D., agrees, noting that meat was rarely the centerpiece of our ancestors' meals as it is today. "We ate a lot of beans, rice, and greens that were only *seasoned* with a little ham hock," she says.

She notes, too, the vast distance between today's Black families and even our recent ancestors when it comes to food preparation. "My grandmother did all her cooking from fresh foods. She snapped her own peas and made black-eyed peas fresh—not from a can," she says. Reliance on processed or refined foods is a recent development.

"I went to a gathering of Black women, and as we were talking about food and cooking habits, I discovered that none of the Black women in their thirties had any idea how to snap beans," she recalls. "Most of them cooked from cans."

In part, this change reflects advances in technology and a growing economy. In the sudden prosperity that followed World War II, growing numbers of Americans, including African-Americans, were able to replace their iceboxes with refrigerators. This meant that women no longer needed fresh ingredients to cook and could reduce the amount of time they spent growing and shopping for food and preparing meals. In the booming postwar economy, they could feed their families processed foods like TV dinners, canned vegetables, and lunch meats, which were unavailable to the previous generations. As a result, they had more time for other activities, including working and leisure.

The Civil Rights revolution affected our cooking and eating habits, too. Before the 1960s, much of the Black community was segregated from Whites, either by law or by custom. That meant Black culture was relatively sheltered from the influence of the dominant culture, which was becoming increasingly convenience-oriented. But as soon as we could motor over to McDonald's without being harassed, African-Americans began to adopt the eating habits that White folks were starting to develop—and it didn't take long for the fast-food companies to realize that Black folks represented an untapped market. We, too, wanted it fast and cheap and in a box.

As a result of adopting a convenience-oriented, "modern" lifestyle, many of us have abandoned—or forgotten—healthful foods and nutritious ways of preparing them. And with the rapidity of technological advancements, we've also left behind the physically active lifestyle that burned off much of the fat and calories we took into our bodies.

What's Being American Got to Do with It?

You can see that the foods that grace our dinner table didn't arrive there overnight. Neither did our diet-related health problems, experts say. Both have developed gradually over the years as our culture has evolved. We're not the only ethnic group whose health has declined after adopting Western ways. Encouraged by tantalizing mass-media images of the "better" life, millions of people around the world have embraced processed, refined foods that are a distant cry from indigenous staples. But these dietary changes have come with a price. Epidemiologists say that when we veer away from our traditional diets, we invite trouble.

"Just look at Native Americans," says nutritionist Lauren Swann. "They suffer from diabetes, hypertension, and obesity—none of which was a problem for them before they abandoned their traditional diet, which was based on corn, beans, vegetables, and some meat."

Or consider Hawaiians, who are more than twice as likely to die from heart disease, cancers, and stroke than are other Americans. Hawaiians are four times as likely to contract an infectious disease and more than six times as likely to die from diabetes, even though the Hawaiian population has been historically healthy.

In a much-respected study, Terry Shintani, M.D., a Hawaiian physician, connected the high incidence of obesity and disease among Hawaiians with their replacement of native foods with a typical Western diet. As processed meals and fast food replaced more traditional favorites, disorders that had rarely afflicted Hawaiians turned into leading killers. By placing his patients on a more traditional diet, Dr. Shintani improved their health and reduced their reliance on medications.

Dr. Coker-Ross cites a prime example of how the White culture has influenced the way people of color eat. When she hired a woman from Ethiopia to help prepare meals in her home, the woman started out frying most of the food.

"As it turned out, before she came to work for me, the woman had worked for an elderly White woman who had taught her to fry," the physician recalls. "But when I told her to just cook the way she would if she were at home [in Ethiopia], she included more fresh vegetables in the meal and relied less on processed foods or frying."

Of course, many processed, refined, fried foods are the very backbone—the "soul"—of soul food. And when you add up the standard American (and African-American) diet, what do you get? Eggs, bacon, and a glass of juice or whole milk in the morning, some meat or cheese between a couple of slices of white bread at noon, and a hunk of meat, some macaroni and cheese, and something green in the evening. It seems harmless and wholesome enough. It's certainly lip-smackin' tasty. But it also adds up to a heaping helping of fat and cholesterol, far too little fiber, and surprisingly too much protein.

"The present American diet, with its emphasis on dairy, meat, fish, chicken, and oils, accounts for 75 percent of our diseases," says Caldwell Esselstyn Jr., M.D., head of thyroid and parathyroid surgery at the Cleveland Clinic Foundation. "Namely, heart disease, stroke, hypertension, adult-onset diabetes, osteoporosis, and cancer of the breast, prostate, colon, and ovary."

And if American cultural trends continue, unless we take some drastic action, it appears that things will get only worse. Americans of all races live in a "toxic food environment," claims Professor Kelly Brownell, a professor of psychology, epidemiology, and public health at Yale University and one of the nation's leading obesity experts, in Nutrition Action Newsletter, a publication of the Center for Science in the Public Interest (CSPI). "Americans have unprecedented access to a poor diet—to high-calorie foods that are widely available, low in cost, heavily promoted, and good tasting. These ingredients produce a predictable, understandable, and inevitable consequence—an epidemic of diet-related diseases."

No wonder it's so hard to eat healthily given our cultural landscape. And it shouldn't surprise you that you have trouble with your weight. The bottom line: We're all ultimately responsible for what we take into our bodies, and we each have to live with the consequences. Still, the fact that Black folks are struggling with weight gain isn't because we're weak and it isn't all our fault. We're fighting an uphill battle against powerful cultural forces—both American and African-American—as well as international businesses whose fortunes depend on our constant consumption of foods and beverages that aren't in our nutritional or biological best interest.

All the more reason we need a diet that's different—an approach to weight-loss that harnesses the power of our minds, bodies, and spirits to develop a healthier lifestyle, a program that helps us overcome the unique combination of cultural forces that have brought us to this crossroad. Good for us that we come from a long line of determined and unbelievably spiritual people—successful ancestor-survivors who overcame obstacles far greater than losing weight. The power of their spirit is part of our cultural legacy and will guide us in our endeavor to develop a more healthy approach to life.

lightenUP

CHAPTER 1

Sow the Seeds for Success

An Overview of the *HealthQuest* 30-Day Weight-Loss Program

When you think of the word "diet" you probably think "temporary"—as in something to help you fit into that *baaad* size 8 (or 18) dress for that fancy holiday party. It's something you do to lose weight. Or perhaps it reminds you of the word "disappointment"; most people find that dieting and disappointment are as close in real life as they are in the dictionary.

But a diet, by definition, is bigger than either one of those thoughts; it's the sum total of everything you eat, every day. That means you've been on a diet from day one. Of course, smothered pork chops and peach cobbler are a far cry from mother's milk and rice cereal. But just because your diet hasn't always been perfect doesn't mean you haven't been on one.

Ideally, your diet changes over the years so that you're taking in the proper nutrients for your age, activity level, and nutrition needs. A teenage girl and a college football player have very different dietary needs. And as they both get older, their diets must change. If that football player keeps shoveling in the steak and potatoes after he's left his shoulder pads behind, he may find himself with extra padding in some other places.

If you're reading this book, maybe your diet has changed too much—or not enough—so that you're gaining more weight than you need for your age, build, and lifestyle. Maybe your doctor has even told you that you need to lose weight. So now you're looking for a diet to lose the extra pounds. The *HealthQuest* 30-Day Weight-Loss Program can help you do that—and much more. It's a healthy, culturally relevant, and holistic method of weight loss that engages your mind and spirit as well as your body. Because it's so comprehensive, you're much more likely to be successful in losing weight and keeping it off for the long haul.

In this chapter, we'll spend some time looking at the concept of diets. You'll learn why most diets aren't worth the paper they're printed on. You'll also learn how your *HealthQuest* 30-Day Weight-Loss Program is different from diets and why this program—with its emphasis on holistic weight loss and culturally relevant foods—succeeds where others fail. And we'll take a look at what you can expect during the course of the thirty days.

Future Shock

Picture a room containing one hundred African-Americans. It's a mixed group—a sample of the typical dieting population: mostly women but a few brothers; young parents and graying seniors; high-school grads along with Ph.D.s. A while ago, each of them chose a different diet and lost twenty-five pounds. This is a happy room; the air is electric with smiles and hugs.

These smiles would surely fade if our one hundred friends could foresee the future. Statistically speaking, if there was a reunion of folks who kept off the weight for two years, the room would hold only ten of the one hundred original dieters. That's right: 90 percent of all dieters who lose twenty-five pounds or more can't keep it off for two years, according to the National Center for Health Statistics.

If there were another reunion of successful dieters after seven years, only two people would show up. Most of the original dieters would have gained back all of their lost weight, and many would actually weigh more than they did originally.

Diets fail. And when they do, it's only natural to blame ourselves. The usual logic that we use is this:

1. This diet works (or else Junie at the beauty shop and Miss Maybelle and her cousin down at the church and half of the rest of the neighborhood wouldn't be raving about it).

2. Unlike Phen-fen and those other dangerous diet schemes, this one is obviously safe (or else the Food and Drug Administration or someone would be warning folks about it).

3. When I followed the diet, I lost some weight at first, but then I stopped losing and actually started gaining some. In the end, those lost pounds flew right back onto my hips (or thighs or belly or butt) faster than I could say "cottage cheese."

4. Conclusion: I must have done something wrong.

And that's where we go astray. Sure, we might not have followed that diet to the letter. We admit it: We may have given ourselves overly generous portions or snuck in an ice-cream sandwich between asparagus spears. But even if you had followed the diet to the letter, it might still have bombed. The reason isn't you. Blame it on: (1) the diet itself; and (2) how the human body reacts when it's deprived of food. Let's take a look at these two crucial issues one at a time. First, we'll take a look at the business of dieting. Then we'll teach you about what your body does when it's confronted with a reduction in calories.

Anatomy of a Diet Plan

A few years ago, Joanna Dwyer, Ph.D., a professor of Nutrition at Tufts University Medical School, was concerned over the rash of unproven diets on the market. So she drew up a list of criteria to help consumers evaluate whether or not a diet was a good deal. The list contained sixteen questions to ask:

1. Is the program safe?
2. Does the plan involve exercise?
3. Is the rate of weight loss reasonable (4 to 8 pounds per month)?
4. Is the diet restrictive?
5. Is the diet nutritionally balanced?
6. Does the diet contain liquid formulas?
7. Does the diet provide appetite suppressants?
8. Can the diet be followed?
9. Does the diet make scientific and common sense?

10. Does it suit the dieter's particular psychological, social, and physiological needs?
11. Does it deal with emotional adjustments to weight loss?
12. Does it include behavioral and environmental modification techniques?
13. Are motivation and support provided to help the dieter assume responsibility for weight loss?
14. Is the cost reasonable? Are special foods, special devices, books, or fees involved?
15. Is there a way to keep the weight off after the program ends?
16. Can the dieter monitor the program?

When Dr. Dwyer tested sixty popular diets against her criteria, forty-two of them flunked outright. Lots of diets that are popular today don't do very well against these questions.

Take the liquid diet—the one where you drink two shakes and eat a sensible meal each day. This one flunks the "scientific and common sense" test. The shakes have lots of vitamins and minerals, but no shake can compensate for the full nutritional spectrum found in real food. And common sense will tell you that drinking two shakes a day gets old fast. You want to *chew* something sometimes and experience a wide variety of flavors and textures. Pretty soon, most people think, "If I so much as see one more shake I may turn into one!" So they ditch the diet to save their sanity—forfeiting any weight loss in the process.

And the meat-lover's diet, the cabbage soup diet, or any other diet that suggests that you consume megadoses of any one type of food, flunks not only the "scientific and common sense" test, but the "nutritionally balanced" test and the "too restrictive" test, too. The meat-lover's diet defies all good advice to steer away from the traditional American diet, which is already too rich in protein, and to make plant foods—beans, grains, vegetables, fruits—the foundation of your meals. And with the weight loss reported on the cabbage soup diet—upward of fifteen pounds in a week—it also fails the "reasonable rate of weight loss" test. Not to mention the fact that we all have our limits; even a rabbit can't eat cabbage forever.

We're not just picking on these three diet plans. The point is, once you start subjecting weight-loss plans to a few basic criteria, lots of them don't hold up. That's the first reason why you shouldn't blame yourself when a diet fails—most diets aren't that great to begin with.

Why We're Different

But the *HealthQuest* 30-Day Weight-Loss Program is different from most diets. With its healthy, balanced, and holistic approach, it holds its own against Dr. Dwyer's sixteen-point list. Here's how:

1. *Is the program safe?* Yes. Ours is designed to be healthy rather than faddish. We're health editors, after all—and we're working with doctors, nutritionists, and health experts to make triple-sure we don't lead you astray. Every bit of advice on these pages is physician-tested and clinically sound. But do check with your doctor before you begin this or any weight-loss plan; you could have a health condition that warrants special attention.

2. *Does the plan involve exercise?* Yes. For reasons we'll explain in chapter 9, the *HealthQuest* 30-Day Weight-Loss Program *cannot work* without physical activity. No ifs, ands, or buts about it. Don't worry—it'll be so enjoyable that you'll wonder how you lived without it. But if you haven't exercised in a while, it's crucial to check with your doc before starting this aspect of your thirty-day program, too.

3. *Is the rate of weight loss reasonable (4 to 8 pounds per month)?* Yes. Researchers say the key to losing permanent pounds is to do it gradually. On the *HealthQuest* 30-Day Weight-Loss Program, you'll learn how to lose one to two pounds of fat per week, four to eight pounds per month. It's a goal that won't feel overwhelming. And you'll be able to repeat the thirty-day cycle as many times as necessary if you want to lose additional weight.

4. *Is the diet restrictive?* Not at all. We know the stresses and joys, the limitations and the satisfactions, of being Black in America. When a faraway daughter comes home to visit, when someone is ailing, when it's time to celebrate—we fire up the oven. Likewise, food seems to ease the strains of dealing with daily stressors—from racism and job pressure to family trouble and loneliness. So we'll provide you with

choices along the way. Not only will we teach you how to craft a weight-loss strategy that's right for you, we'll provide you with two weeks' worth of healthy menus, along with thirty-one delectable soul food recipes created by noted nutritionist Dr. Goulda Downer—foods like Finger-Licking Curried Chicken, Scrumptious Red Beans and Rice, Savory Potato Salad, and Great Big Biscuits. All of the recipes are low in fat, calories, sodium, and cholesterol. And we'll even help you make friends with a few foods you may not know about.

5. *Is the diet nutritionally balanced?* You bet it is. The program contains all of the protein, carbohydrates, fats, vitamins, and minerals that you need for a vibrant, active life.

6. *Does the diet contain liquid formulas?* No. You can make a low-fat fruit shake if you'd like, but whole foods are the backbone of this diet. The emphasis is on foods that are minimally processed, that contain few additives, and that resonate with our ancestral culture.

7. *Does the diet provide appetite suppressants?* No, this program doesn't rely on appetite-curbing pills or on pharmaceutical formulas. The delicious whole foods you'll enjoy in this diet do contain plenty of fiber, which acts as a natural appetite suppressant by helping you feel pleasantly full.

8. *Can the diet be followed?* The *HealthQuest* 30-Day Weight-Loss Program is straightforward as well as immensely educational. You know the old African proverb, "If you give a man a fish, he'll eat for a day; if you teach him how to fish, he'll eat for a lifetime"? Well, we'll teach you the reasoning behind the advice and recommendations in this book so you'll be able to follow the program as well as make informed choices on your own. We'll empower you with the information you need to protect yourself from unhealthy but widely accepted habits that are part of both American and African-American culture. And as we told you earlier, we'll give you choices so you can adjust as circumstances demand.

9. *Does it make scientific and common sense?* It makes the *most* sense. Our program is consistent with two sets of expert advice—on weight loss specifically and healthy living generally. To lose weight and keep it off, experts say you need to eat fewer total calories (especially fat calories) and increase your amount and level of exercise. To build a

healthy, strong body: eat less protein, fewer fats, and less refined sweets, and more whole grains, beans, vegetables, and fruits. That's the scientific consensus these days, but it also makes common sense—it's essentially the same type of diet our ancestors thrived on for generations.

10. *Does it suit the dieter's particular psychological, social, and physiological needs?* The *HealthQuest* 30-Day Weight-Loss Program is a holistic plan. That means it's not just a list of foods you can eat and foods you can't. It caters to your physiological, psychological, emotional, and spiritual needs—a total package that's designed by African-Americans for African-Americans.

11. *Does it deal with emotional adjustments to weight loss?* Absolutely. Your body is intertwined with your emotions, your soul, your spirit—all of your component parts—so it's pointless to offer a weight-loss program that modifies your diet without addressing the mental and emotional reasons you eat. So, at the end of each chapter, you'll find "Think It Through" exercises to help you examine issues, such as why you eat the way you eat and your feelings about exercise, and "For Your Spirit" exercises, to inspire you and to help you overcome mental and physical obstacles to success. We'll also help you mentally adjust to the changes you'll experience and help you figure out what to do if you don't lose as much weight as you expect.

12. *Does it include behavioral- and environmental-modification techniques?* The "Think It Through" exercises at the end of every chapter are designed to help you understand why you eat and exercise the way you do, pinpoint what you need to do to change, then ease into a new way of doing things. That can include keeping new foods in the pantry, getting out of the house for a little power-walking through the mall, and other environmental changes. We also anticipate challenges to maintaining weight and offer suggestions on how to manage them.

13. *Are motivation and support provided to help the dieter assume responsibility for weight loss?* This book provides plenty of motivation and support, in the form of specific tips on how to accomplish the suggestions we make and inspirational pep talks to get you revved up to do it. But as anyone who's ever tried to quit smoking or do more exercise or give up doughnuts knows, lifestyle changes are always easier if you take them on with a friend. So, if you know a buddy who's trying to lose weight and be healthier, by all means, invite them along for the ride so you can give each other mutual support. There's also a 30-Day Weight-Loss Program Room on the *HealthQuest* website (www.healthquestmag.com) where you can find tools and information to support your weight-loss efforts.

14. *Is the cost reasonable? Are special foods, special devices, books, or fees involved?* There are no special devices or fees, and the foods probably aren't all that different from the ones you already enjoy. As for the price tag, whole foods can cost more than processed, refined foods, and fresh foods can cost more than frozen or canned. But think of it as an investment in your health. Anyway, we're talking small potatoes compared to the hundreds of dollars it can cost to sign up for those fancy franchise diet plans—or the health-care costs you'll rack up if you get sick.

15. *Is there a way to keep the weight off after the program ends?* You don't regain your lost weight because you never stop your new eating and exercise plan! The *HealthQuest* 30-Day Weight-Loss Program is a lot different from any other diet you've tried because it's designed to help you develop healthful practices that will turn into lifelong habits. As long as you stick with the lifestyle changes you learn during the first thirty days, you should be able to maintain your new weight. But if you want to lose more, just repeat the program.

16. *Can the dieter monitor the program?* No problem. Our weight-loss plan is definitely results-oriented. We'll teach you how to look at weight loss in thirty-day increments. Then we'll provide you with handy tools and worksheets to measure your progress. Tools to help you calculate your healthiest weight, set healthy weight-loss goals for each thirty-day cycle, identify the right number of calories to consume each day, and educate you about healthier foods to substitute for the ones that cause the scale to tip upward. We'll also provide places for you to chart your progress so you can see how you are doing. Or you can use the tried-and-true: Check yourself out in the mirror!

So there you have it. When you add it all up, the *HealthQuest* 30-Day Weight-Loss Program satisfies every one of the criteria for safe and effective diet plans. Consider this the first day of a whole lifetime of good health. Here's a quick look at the journey you're about to take.

An Overview of *Lighten Up*

The first section of this book helps you get in the right frame of mind for the challenging work you're about to do. In this section, we'll spend a lot of time talking about food. We'll start by taking note of your personal food choices and preferences, and your fitness routines and habits—but we won't judge them as good or bad, nor will we tell you what you can and cannot do: We know how important it is to have choices and we know how much pleasure food provides. For now, you'll just document your habits so that later you can identify for yourself those habits you want to change.

Next, we'll teach you how to eat for optimum energy, nutrition, and health. We believe that the more you understand about the relationship between food and your body, the more empowered you will feel to make choices that will help you stay healthy and lose weight—and the less burdensome those healthy choices will feel. After reading this information, you may even begin to identify for yourself some ways you'd like to change your diet. In this section, we'll also examine African-Americans' cultural relationship to food, self-image, and weight. We'll look at the many reasons we eat, as well as the impact that our food choices are having on our health. Finally, we'll introduce you to a menu of techniques to help you cut calories from your diet—choices you can tailor to your lifestyle, habits, and food preferences, and still lose weight.

The second section of *Lighten Up* focuses on exercise. When most people think about losing weight, they focus entirely on what they eat, but eating right is just half the battle. When it comes to shaping a sleek, healthy new body, exercise is your secret ally. No healthy weight-loss plan is complete—nor can it be successful in the long term—without a fitness component. So, in the second section, you'll discover the joy of moving your body in wonderful new ways. We'll help you do it gradually, step by step, in a way that feels challenging but not overwhelming, and is definitely enjoyable. You'll learn valuable information on stretching, aerobic exercise, and strength training—the three components of physical fitness that will speed up your metabolism and help you keep weight off. At the end of the section, we'll introduce you to the 7-Day *HealthQuest* Workout, the optimum exercise program for losing weight.

In the final section of the book, you'll take stock of your progress, assess your success and plan your next moves. Could be that you have a few more pounds you'd like to lose. If so, we'll help you make adjustments so you can start the thirty-day weight-loss cycle again. Maybe you've reached your weight-loss goal and want to make sure that you maintain it. In either case, in this section you will find several important weight-loss tools, including worksheets to help you record your progress, pages where you can keep notes, and the calorie count and nutritional information for many common foods.

And there's a huge bonus at the back of the book: recipes that transform traditional African-American favorites into healthful foods that fit your lifestyle and tastes—without the fat, calories, and cholesterol that soul food tends to have. These fresh new recipes—developed by a Black nutritionist, Goulda Downer, Ph.D.—include mouthwatering chicken and fish dishes, savory beans, and delicious greens—all foods familiar in down-home, soul food, and Caribbean cooking. You'll love the fantastic flavors, the savory seasonings, and the colorful celebration of our culinary culture. You'll hardly even know you're dieting. (Don't wait; flip back to page 258 right now.)

A Word to the Wise

Allow us to offer a few words of advice before you delve into the rest of this book. First, don't skip the "Think It Through" or "For Your Spirit" exercises at the end of each chapter. They're designed to prepare you for what's to come, to make you strong as you begin and as you continue your *HealthQuest* 30-Day Weight-Loss Program. The idea here is that permanent weight loss isn't just about shedding pounds—you also need to shed a "fat mentality." This book focuses on the mental and spiritual side of maintaining not just a healthy weight but also maintaining a balanced approach to daily life.

And please, don't just focus on the dietary parts of the book and ignore the exercise chapters. It's vital that you get moving—not just so that your weight-loss efforts can be more effective, but so that you can be healthier overall. Numerous studies show there's no substitute for exercise — especially if you want to lose weight and to keep it off.

Once you've read through the second section of the book and have started to exercise, choose a day when you want to combine the dietary changes with exercise and start your *HealthQuest* 30-Day Weight-Loss Program. Make that Day 1 of your thirty-day program, and follow the guidelines for each of the next twenty-nine days. We know that by Day 30, you'll be happier, saner, more peaceful, more whole—and, in all likelihood, measurably lighter! If you want to lose more weight, just start the thirty-day cycle all over again. In either case, we hope you continue to practice these healthy lifestyle habits.

 Get the Green Light from Your Doctor!

Before starting any health and fitness program, or undertaking any dietary changes or exercise regimen, *see your doctor*. Get a thorough physical exam that includes tests for blood sugar, cholesterol level, vitamin deficiencies, or any other consideration that may affect your diet or your health. If your doctor knows you're engaged in a weight-loss program, he or she will know what to look for. For example, if you're diabetic, you'll want to make sure you're eating regular meals to keep your blood sugar regulated. We want you to start this program with no unforeseen obstacles and to be able to sustain the program without setbacks, so go see your health-care practitioner and get the green light.

Think It Through

What's your diet history? If you're like many of us, you've been on and off diets all your adult life—maybe longer. The diets you've tried may be different, but if you're reading this book, that means the result was ultimately the same: You regained weight.

Think back on all the diets you've done and ask yourself the following questions. Jot down the answers in a notebook that will become your Food and Fitness Diary (more on that in chapter 2).

- What was the basis of the diet?
- How long did you stay on the diet?
- What was your weight-loss goal (how many pounds and in what time frame)? How much weight did you lose?
- What caused you to go off the diet? Did you meet your goal or did you quit for some reason?
- How did you feel physically while you were on the diet? Hungry? Weak? Light-headed? Energetic?
- How did you feel mentally? Emotionally? Were you in any kind of life transition—divorce, moving, new job, death of a loved one?
- Did you exercise regularly while you were dieting?
- Were you able to follow the diet to the letter? Did you "cheat" often?

Now look at your list. You may see some patterns emerge: Perhaps you may always start a diet when things around you are chaotic. Maybe family obligations tempt you to cheat. Maybe your diets have left you mentally or physically drained, so it's harder and harder to get motivated. By looking at your personal diet history, you can more wisely approach the thirty-day program you're about to begin, taking into account your own tendencies and being aware of the ways in which your approach to this diet should be different.

For Your Spirit

Any experienced gardener knows that a lot of work goes into a garden before beautiful flowers and plants appear. Much of this work takes place in the fall, when there's a chill in the air, the flowers from the previous season have died and turned brown, and bulbs for the next year have yet to be planted. There's no glamour in this part of a gardener's work. But a smart gardener will use compost and refuse from the previous season to bring life to the new season coming.

An inexperienced gardener, on the other hand, may appreciate the beauty of bright begonias or the fragrance of freesias, but she has little appreciation for the amount of effort that goes into a garden's creation. Come April, she may head to the garden store and pick up some bulbs that should have been planted in the fall. Or she may purchase pots of plants and not know that where she lives there's likely to be a late frost that will kill her new plants. Our amateur is likely to experience the expense, pain, and frustration that comes from not having prepared for the work that was to come. She may even feel like a failure.

Now, before she begins, our smart gardener does a lot of planning. First, she makes sure she has the tools she needs to do her work. She has gloves, shovels, spades, and trowels at her disposal. She prepares the ground, which may involve digging up and aerating the entire garden or just a small part of it. Our smart gardener may sow her plants indoors, in small pots or trays, so that they are protected from the winter and can develop a strong root system before they are planted in the spring. She conditions the soil with mulch, compost, or manure, and has a strategy for dealing with pests—slugs, weeds, and a variety of vermin—beginning in the fall and throughout the growing season. How does our smart gardener know all this? Because she was once an amateur, but she learned from her mistakes.

So, too, should you as you approach your weight-loss to ensure you'll succeed. Rather than feeling discouraged and frustrated by the limited success you experienced in the past, figure out how you can use the wisdom you've accumulated through your prior efforts to prepare you to attain your goals this time around. Now that you've taken inventory of your previous weight-loss efforts in the "Think It Through" exercise above, it's a good time to consider the ways you'd like this effort to be different.

Just like our smart gardener, a person who is most likely to experience weight-loss success starts her program with the proper tools. Take a moment to pull out your diary and make a list of the tools that will help you with your weight-loss effort.

The most important tool is a willing spirit. Are you feeling up to the conscious effort that losing weight requires? If so, you're starting out on the right foot. But if not, there's no need to get down on yourself. Remember: For everything there is a season, a time, and a place under the sun. Our experienced gardener would never plant flowers in Chicago in December. Nor should you begin a weight-loss program if you're not ready to do the work or your environment doesn't support you.

If, for instance, you're overwhelmed at work, your kids are having problems, or you're in a bad relationship, you've got enough going on; you may not have enough energy to be successful at losing weight right now. And that's okay. Like our experienced gardener who plants her seeds in trays she nurtures indoors over the winter, this may be a time to take smaller steps. Merely reading this book is a great move in the right direction. Even if you read the book and start to implement only minor changes in your diet or commit to taking the stairs more often, you're taking the small steps that add up to big changes. Know that every little bit helps. Losing and maintaining weight is a lifelong process. God willing, you'll have plenty more time to get it right.

Or maybe you're conflicted about losing weight. You'd like to be slimmer but aren't quite sure you want to do the work. Don't start just to set yourself up to fail. Wait until you feel differently. Perhaps as you read this book and complete the exercises, you'll get your spirit in better shape. After a few chapters—or even after you read the book through one time —you may feel motivated and ready to start. But whether you're ready, conflicted, or need to wait to get started, take the time to complete the exercises and write about how you feel. Sometimes writing about things makes them clearer for us, and we feel more empowered to make things change.

In addition to being spiritually ready, this is a good time to think about some other tools. Now make a list of the physical tools to help you on your weight-loss journey. Do it right now in your diary. Perhaps you saw a bunch of vegetable steamers on the clearance rack at the dollar store. You're going to be eating more vegetables soon, and steaming is a wonderful way to prepare them. Go ahead and get one now. You may have read about a healthy-cooking class at the community college or adult education center in your area—or an ethnic cooking class at a local restaurant. What a fantastic way to add excitement to your cooking reper-toire and a wonderful investment in a healthy new you.

Maybe your sneakers are a bit run over and it's time to pick up a new pair. Or you'd feel more comfortable exercising if you ran out to the dis-count store and purchased a larger sweatsuit. If you've been planning to join the gym or to take yoga at your local Y, sign up now. All of these are appropriate tools that will support your desire to lose weight. This is the time to invest in yourself. Even small monetary investments can have a big payoff.

It's also time for you to cultivate the soil and prepare your environ-ment. Make a list of all the things you can do to make your life as happy and as positive as possible. A positive environment builds upon itself in the very same way that negativity snowballs. By creating small but posi-tive changes throughout your life, you create fertile soil in which to plant your aspirations to lose weight.

If you're like many people, you feel better about yourself if you engage in some sort of regular devotion. Maybe it's prayer, maybe it's meditation, or going to church on Sunday, volunteering, or contemplatively working in the garden. Whatever it is, now's the time to start—or to start again. (We always have the opportunity to start again or to make different choices.) Some people feel better about themselves when they get up early to get a jump on the day; night owls feel better when they stay up late. Either way, pick a quiet time to engage in introspection and do the exercises you'll find throughout the book. Maybe you've wanted to start a walking club. It's time to call your friends over for your first meeting. Perhaps you like to write, draw, play flag football, read, do calligraphy, rebuild automobile engines, sketch, play in the basketball league, paint, sing, cook, work in your wood shop, go to the movies, paint your finger-nails, figure out new hairstyles, sew, meditate, fix things around the house, garden, burn fragrant candles, listen to inspirational music, spend time with your makeup, hike, sky dive, in-line skate, or sit on your porch swing. Whatever it is that you love to do, write it down on your list and begin to do it more often. Remember: When you do things that make you feel good about yourself, you create fertile ground for other positive actions.

Now for the hard part—clearing the weeds, dealing with pests and other naysayers. Perhaps you feel better about yourself when your home is neat and you've cleared the clutter. If so, take a weekend to clean it thoroughly and get your house in order. Most of us feel better when we're on top of our finances and pay our bills on time. To the extent that you can do this, do so as often as possible.

And you don't need us to tell you who the naysayers are in your environment. But now's the time to develop a strategy for dealing with them. If you've been thinking about ending a negative friendship, maybe you can do it now. It may require a conversation or maybe you can just let them drift away. If your best friend is always trying to shove another plate full of fried chicken wings in your face, perhaps it's time you stop eating with him and start doing something else with him, instead.

It's also important to begin to think about how you'll handle the people who may want to sabotage you. You know the kind of people—the ones who like to wave a piece of coconut cake under your nose just to see if you'll give in, the ones who joke about your weight-loss efforts, the people who will tell you the stories about all the folks they know who gained back all the weight they lost. As you probably already know, not everyone is going to be happy that you're losing weight. Some friends or family members may feel threatened that you'll lose weight and leave them behind. Others may lose their feeling of being better than you if they can't criticize you for being heavy. Or maybe your relationship with them is focused around food.

Some of the people who are most upset may be the people you're closest to. They may want you to stay just as you are. You'll need a strategy to deal with each of these types of people. So right now, in the privacy of your diary, begin to develop ideas about how you'll deal with them. Unlike the last time, you may decide not to announce to everyone that you've decided to begin a weight-loss program. Your decision to lose weight may be something you choose to keep to yourself or to share with only a chosen few. Remember, smart gardeners sow some seeds in small trays indoors. And all this preparation helps create the conditions that will ultimately yield a beautiful harvest.

CHAPTER 2

An Essential Tool for Sound Mind, Body, and Spirit

Your Food and Fitness Diary

A s you learned in chapter 1, any reputable weight-loss program will encourage you to improve your eating habits and to adopt some kind of exercise routine. Now, depending upon who you are, that may mean that you need to make significant changes to your diet or perhaps just clip a couple of calories here and there; to begin exercising for the first time in your life or adapt an already existing routine. But before you can seriously start to think about making lifestyle changes, you first need to assess where you're at—look at what you're currently eating and how much exercise you're now getting.

So, before you count a single calorie or walk a block, we're going to ask you to make a quick run to the store and pick up a notebook. Choose a notebook that isn't going to get torn to bits or have pages falling out. It should be small enough that you can carry it back and forth between your home and work, but large enough for you to write your thoughts in. This will become your Food and Fitness Diary. We want you to use this diary also to record the answers to the "Think It Through" and "For Your Spirit" exercises at the end of each chapter. You may also want to use it to record your personal thoughts, especially as they relate to losing weight. But first, you'll need it to do a bit of "homework"—an easy two-part self-assessment exercise in which you don't have to change a thing you eat and you don't even have to start exercising. We simply want you to use your diary to record what you eat and your level of activity for an entire week.

Self-Assessment I: Track Your Food

We take eating for granted, so much so that most folks aren't even conscious of what they're eating—or when or why. In some cases, people eat less than they imagine, but if you find you need to lose weight, you may be eating more than you realize. Or perhaps your diet isn't quite as balanced as you think. Maybe one little food weakness (needing a cookie or two before bed every night) or eating habit (skipping breakfast, eating late dinners) is the secret to your extra pounds. Well, whatever your weakness is, we're here to help you find it and begin to address it.

For the first part of our two-part exercise, just pick a starting day and write down everything you eat and drink for one week. Everything—that means all meals, snacks, drinks, even water. Include *everything*—even a few chips you took from your son's bag or the spoonful of ice cream you ate, as well as significant condiments like the cream in your coffee, salad dressing or mayonnaise, and jelly, butter, or margarine.

Now, don't try to be perfect and write down only the foods you feel good about eating. We want you to take stock of where you *really* are. (Remember what your teachers told you: If you don't know your past, you're bound to repeat it—and we're trying to create a new future!) List each food on a separate line moving down the page (see the diary example that follows). Also, along with each entry write down the following:

- *The time of day.* Be specific (not just "morning" or "evening") but "Around 1:30" or "6:00." Don't worry if you don't have it down to the minute, though.
- *Your location.* Are you at the dinner table, in the car, at your desk, in front of the television?
- *Who's there.* Are you alone? With your family? Having drinks with your pals?
- *Your mood.* Are you angry with your boss? Celebrating some victory? Frustrated with your spouse?

When you complete this activity for an entire week, you're done. There's nothing else you need to do right now. We'll tell you how to analyze your Food and Fitness Diary in chapter 4, to help you personalize the best program suited for you.

Reminders

• Don't worry about what's on those pages right now; that doesn't matter. Just the fact that you're writing things down is probably going to make you eat a bit more conscientiously, but don't fake it. It may make you feel good to see nice balanced meals listed—but if that's not your normal food routine, it's not going to help you figure out your food weaknesses. There's no good or bad, no right or wrong at this point. The most important thing is to make sure that you have a complete record of what's going into your mouth. Remember: No one is going to see this diary but you.

• Don't whip out your notebook in the office cafeteria. No need for everyone in the world to know what you're doing. No, it's not a big secret. But your weight—and your weight loss—are private affairs, and you don't need the office skeptic or your forever-joking girlfriend scrutinizing your efforts. Wait until you have a minute to yourself to write things down— *just don't forget to do it.*

• Review your food diary at the end of the day. Visualize your day and picture each time you ate something. If you forgot to jot something down, now's the time to fill in the blanks.

Here's an example of what your diet diary might look like:

Monday		
	8:15 a.m.	*1 large blueberry muffin*
		1 pat of butter
		1 coffee with cream and sugar
		half glass of water

Had to be at work early so ate at my desk, feeling anxious about important staff meeting.

10:30 a.m.   1 package of cheese crackers
              cup of coffee with cream and sugar
After staff meeting, went to snack machine with Lillian. Wanted something to tide me over until lunch.

1:30 p.m.   9 chicken nuggets with BBQ sauce
              large fries
              soda
Trying to finish project, so sent Al to pick up lunch. Ate at my desk.

4:00 p.m.   diet soda
Something to keep me going for the rest of the afternoon and to be pepped up for rush hour.

7:00 p.m.   2 slices meatloaf, no gravy
              mashed potatoes, pat of margarine
              carrots
              1 slice bread
              soda
Planned to broil chicken, but Ron wanted meatloaf. Dinner was late. I did eat a few Ritz crackers while fixing dinner. About 10.

9:30 p.m.   corn chips and salsa
Watching TV. Feeling tired. Still a little annoyed with Ron.

11:00 p.m.   three tablespoons frozen yogurt
              1 glass water
Standing in front of freezer. Needed something sweet before bed. Another meeting tomorrow. Dreading that.

Self-Assessment II: Monitor Your Activity

Like the food-tracking component of the exercise, this second part is also designed to help you determine where you are—but with regard to your current activity level. You'll get a sense of how active you already are, so that when it's time to begin your new fitness program, you'll have a starting place from which to set goals.

Use a separate section of your Food and Fitness Diary to record your activity level for one week. Don't worry—this is going to be easier than it may sound.

Don't feel you need to whip out your diary and scribble a note every time you bend down to tie your shoes. Just take a few minutes at lunch and the end of each day to record roughly how much time you've spent doing active and inactive things. You're looking for activities that keep you constantly moving. And we're not just talking about working out; mowing the lawn counts, as does raking leaves, walking your baby in the stroller, and doing moderately heavy housework, like mopping the floor. Of course, speed-walking is more strenuous and, therefore, burns more calories and strengthens your heart more than gardening does, but if it keeps you in motion, gardening counts. Identify these activities and round them off to the nearest fifteen minutes (make sure you don't round everything upward or you'll overestimate your activity level and the number of calories you're burning). You don't have to account for every single moment, but try to account for all twenty-four hours, give or take a quarter-hour or two.

You may prefer to record your activity level during the same week as you record everything you eat and drink, or maybe you'd rather do these exercises separately in different weeks. Choose whatever works best for you.

Don't worry about how much or how little activity you're engaged in. The goal in this exercise is to record what you do—not to evaluate it. Just jot down your daily activities like this young office worker did below.

What I Did	When I Did It	Total time
Dressing, eating breakfast	7:00–7:45 a.m.	0.75 hr.
Driving to work	7:45–8:15 a.m.	0.50 hr.
Work at desk	8:30–noon	3.50 hrs.
Lunch at Fish Shack (drove)	noon–1:00 p.m.	1 hr.
Work at desk	1:00–5:00 p.m.	4 hrs.

Driving home	5:15–5:45 p.m	0.50 hr.
Change clothes, lie down for rest	5:45–6:30 p.m.	0.75 hr.
Cook, have dinner with Bill	6:30–8:00 p.m.	1.50 hrs.
Watching TV	8:00–11:00 p.m.	3 hrs.
Sleeping	11:00–7:00 a.m.	8 hrs.

What It All Means: Evaluating Your Eating and Activity Level

Later, in chapter 4, we'll give you some valuable information on the program choices available to you, based on what you learn from tracking your foods for the week. (We guarantee that the tracking exercise will prove valuable time and again in informing you of your preferences and eating details that you may not even be conscious of.) You'll be able to draw conclusions that will steer you to the most appropriate thirty-day program to fit your own needs, food preferences, and lifestyle. But for now, let's focus on your activity.

After you've monitored your activity for a week, choose a day of the week from your Food and Fitness Diary that shows a typical amount of activity for you. It can be the same day as the one you chose to evaluate your diet, or a different day. Now answer these questions:

1. How much time did you spend lying down, sitting, driving, or being still?
   - 18 hours or more
   - 16–18 hours
   - 14–16 hours
   - 12–14 hours
   - 10–12 hours
   - 8–10 hours
   - 8 hours or less

2. How much time did you spend walking, climbing stairs, or doing something active as part of your daily routine? Include your work, if it

is strenuous enough to get your heart pumping for more than fifteen minutes at a time. (Sorry, being on your feet all day doesn't count; you've got to be constantly moving.)

- 1 hour or more
- 30 minutes to 1 hour
- 15–30 minutes
- less than 15 minutes

3. Did you participate in other exercise on the day you selected? If so, for how long.

No.

Yes. For _____ minutes.

Setting Exercise Goals

First of all, if you're getting more than thirty minutes of activity each day, give yourself a hand. Experts suggest that if you can accumulate at least thirty minutes a day of moderately intense physical activity five or more days a week, you'll experience the health benefits of exercise. Any exercise is better for you than getting none at all. But if you're trying to lose weight, you'll want to err on the side of doing more exercise than less—and more vigorous exercise, at that.

Remember: If you cut an extra 500 calories a day, you'll lose a pound each week. The healthiest—and most manageable—way to do that is to cut 250 calories from your diet and expend 250 calories exercising.

Later in the book, we'll teach you more about the relationship between activity level and calorie consumption, but to give you an example, here's a list of exercises you can do to burn 250 calories.

Does this list look overwhelming to you or not as bad as you thought? If it looks overwhelming, remember that you can start off slowly and build up. You can even exercise in short spurts, like fifteen minutes in the morning and fifteen minutes after work. And as we mentioned above, other activities like housework can count. In any case, please stay open-minded to the idea of increasing your activity level. We'll teach you more about it in the next several chapters. We'll even give you a fitness program designed by a fitness expert. Eventually you may get so excited about how

Activity	Minutes of exercise to burn 250 calories			
	125 lb.	150 lb.	175 lb.	200 lb.
Aerobic dance (moderate)	32 min.	27 min.	23 min.	20 min.
Aerobic dance (vigorous)	21 min.	18 min.	15 min.	13 min.
Bicycling, 19 mph	26 min.	22 min.	19 min.	16 min.
Running, 7.5 mph	21 min.	18 min.	15 min.	13 min.
Swimming, 45 yd/min.	34 min.	29 min.	25 min.	22 min.
Walking, 3.5 mph	57 min.	48 min.	41 min.	36 min.
Walking, 4.5 mph	42 min.	35 min.	30 min.	26 min.

you feel and look as a result of exercise that you find yourself wanting to do even more.

For now, just start moving. Do whatever you want to or can do, getting a little more active each day. Walk to the corner, take the stairs, stand when you could be sitting, walk to the TV to change the channel, rake instead of using the leaf-blower. All of these activities burn calories. Burn a couple here and a couple there. Pretty soon they start adding up.

Think It Through

Everyone has different reasons for wanting to lose weight. Some people want to shed some pounds because they have a new love interest in their life. Others because their children or significant other has begun to express concern. Still others because they want to avoid developing a serious medical problem.

Whether or not any of these descriptions apply to you, you are certainly dieting for a reason. Let's take a look at what you have in mind. Take out your Food and Fitness Diary and write down your answers to the following questions:

- Why do I want to lose weight?
- How much weight do I want to lose?
- Over what period of time did I gain this weight?
- Was anything new or unusual going on when I gained this weight? Did it just accumulate over time?

- How will I benefit by losing weight?
- Is there anyone else in my life who wants me to lose weight? If so, what's in it for them?
- Am I trying to lose weight for myself or for others?

Then compare the answers to these questions to the answers to the "Think It Through" questions in chapter 1. Do any patterns emerge? If you identify any patterns or common themes, make sure to write about them. Is there anything you can do differently this time to avoid prior pitfalls and make your efforts more likely to succeed?

For Your Spirit

If you've read any of the new self-help books that abound these days, you've probably seen the word "affirmation" a hundred times. Or you may have spoken an affirmation of faith in your church. An affirmation is a statement, spoken as if it were already true, designed to reinforce something that you want to recognize or realize in your life.

Affirmations capture the power of the spoken word. The Bible says God spoke into the universe and created the world. Even modern physics can prove that words have transformative powers. Scientists can demonstrate that when we speak, the sound creates a vibration that keeps rippling endlessly, as if we'd thrown a pebble into a still pond. No wonder we know to keep our distance when someone's giving off negative vibes.

Still, you may think it silly to say "I live a life of abundance and prosperity" when your credit cards are maxed out and your rent check just bounced. But the idea is that if you say something enough, you'll reprogram your thinking and develop behaviors that support your new thoughts. At the same time, when you alter your language about yourself, you signal to the universe that you're willing to change. If you're attentive, you'll see how quickly your world begins to support you and changes begin to manifest in your life.

Yet while many of us are familiar with affirmations, we may have learned to make negative ones: "I'm sick and tired of being overweight," instead of the more positive: "I am moving toward a healthy weight for me." Or, "I don't want to fail again," instead of, "I am successful."

But the more we dwell on and speak about the things we *don't* want to happen, the more power we give to those negative thoughts. Remember, our words send energy rippling throughout the universe. And by speaking and thinking negative thoughts over and over, we carve them so deeply into our subconscious that we become resistant to the very changes we want to make.

Those of us—and there are many—who are in the habit of speaking negative affirmations need to begin to retrain our minds. We want to stop our thoughts from heading into familiar negative ruts and give them a new and positive path to follow. It's the only way to reach a different destination.

To do that, we need to make *positive* affirmations that focus our energy on what we *do* want to happen rather than what we *don't* want to happen. By changing the things we believe and say about ourselves, we not only empower ourselves to change our behavior but we ask the Creator to give us a hand.

Find a quiet time and place, sit down with a pen and paper, and practice writing positive affirmations. Write, "I love the fact that I am resilient and always willing to give myself another chance," instead of, "Every time I try, I fail." "I have a round, kind face and a friendly smile," rather than, "I have a fat face, double chin, and a gap between my teeth."

First practice making positive affirmations about any subject you choose. Then focus on affirmations that support your desire to lose weight. If you're having trouble thinking of positive affirmations or are at a loss about how to turn your negative thinking and speaking into a more positive form, take some pointers from the list below.

Old Negative Affirmation	New Positive Affirmation
I'm embarrassed about how I look.	I am becoming comfortable in my new body.
I need to lose weight.	I'm creating a healthy and slender body.
I hate my job.	I'm drawing new and exciting work to me.
I can't seem to stop nibbling.	I am powerful and am putting down this snack.
I am sick and tired of being fat.	I am enjoying becoming healthy.

I hate having such a large behind.	I love my sexy hips, thighs, and behind.
I can't make all these changes.	I am changing myself with joy, ease, and grace.
This is a waste of time and won't work.	I accept new ideas and challenges in my life.
I can't do this.	Through God all things are possible.

As you write your affirmations, you may find it useful to think of them as seeds you are preparing to plant in your subconscious. In nature, seeds contain much of the biological material and all of the genetic information they need to develop into a full-grown plant. The same is true with an affirmation. Words that seem hollow when you first write or say them have the potential to turn into a dream come true.

Focus on a couple of affirmations you'd like to plant in your subconscious to help you change your diet, start to exercise, and create a healthier body, mind, and spirit. Be bold; you don't have to share them with anyone else. Your affirmations should reflect whatever goal or dream you may have—however far it might seem to be from your reality. And don't worry about which affirmations to select and which to set aside; you can incorporate the others at any point along the way. Write your affirmations on a list you can carry around with you.

Now practice saying them out loud, as if they were happening right now. Imagine the vibration of the sound and breath of your positive words rippling outward, touching other things and people, shifting things in the universe so that everything you need in order to accomplish your goals can start moving toward you—remember that both faith and physics have proven this power. Allow yourself to imagine the wonderful coincidences that are about to take place. Maybe a new neighbor will need a partner to work out with, perhaps you'll "stumble across" a healthy new restaurant on your way to work or your bus driver will just "happen" to mention that they're building a new gym in the shopping center you pass on the ride home. All these "coincidences" are God at work, so be alert for them; they're everywhere.

Make an agreement with yourself that you're going to repeat your affirmations every day. Don't worry about following any particular regimen; you're going to start by doing what feels right for you. Some people repeat the same affirmation as often as they can until it feels real. Others believe you need to repeat an affirmation for twenty-one days before it becomes a habit. Some repeat the same thought upon arising and at bed-time. Still others have a different affirmation for morning, noon, and night. You can say an affirmation as a prayer before your meals. Or you can say it all day and write it twenty times at night. Do whatever feels most comfortable for you.

At *HealthQuest* we know that saying affirmations is a spiritual act, but that doesn't mean it can't also be a lot of fun. You don't have to repeat them in a quiet and reverent manner, you can sit in your car, roll up the windows (or not!), and shout affirmations at the top of your lungs while you're driving down the highway. You can change the words to your favorite song and make it your affirmation tune. Sing to yourself while you're at work or when you're bathing in the shower. Create an affirma-tion dance to accompany your new affirmation jam, then embarrass your children by doing it when their friends come over. Do your dance as you prepare your dinner. Hum your song as you take your healthy lunch out of your brown paper bag. Feel your heart flickering to life, your blood pick up tempo, your youthful exuberance again.

Continue to speak your affirmations as lovingly as if they were seeds. Allow them to grow in the fertile soil of your own self-love, nourish them with a healthy diet, and water them with exercise. Before long, you will push through the dark earth of your own fear and resistance. You will begin to see and feel positive changes sprouting in your body, mind, and spirit. These changes will build upon themselves and one positive change will lead to another just as thick branches create new twigs. When people say they notice a change in you, you can smile and tell them you're turn-ing over a new leaf. Now the same affirmations you used to repeat with-out a sense of conviction will begin to feel real, the roots of your new beliefs will grow deep and strong, and new behaviors will become healthy habits. You will bask in the sunlight of your own success, your body will begin to move with comfort and ease, and you will shed your old, negative beliefs as gracefully as a tree sheds leaves.

CHAPTER 3

Laying Your Foundation

The Fundamentals of Nutrition

You are about to embark upon one of the most important lifestyle changes you could ever hope to undertake—the process of learning to care for and nourish yourself to achieve and maintain your optimum weight. At the same time, you'll be tending to your health. Like any other lifestyle change you may choose to make, it's helpful to think of the process in terms of a journey. In this case, your destination is the state where you've achieved—and sustained—your desired weight and are experiencing the corresponding health benefits. But you don't get there overnight. In the words of an ancient proverb: The journey of a thousand miles begins with a single step.

So, let's start at the very beginning. In this chapter, we'll review the fundamentals of good nutrition. We'll tell you up front that there's a lot of heavy information here, but it will be the base of knowledge that you'll use for the rest of your life. We feel it's important to share these nutrition facts because they will empower you to make healthy decisions about food choices and weight loss long after you've put down this book. As they say, knowledge is power—and those who don't understand their past are doomed to repeat it. Find yourself a quiet environment with no distractions. You might also want to ask the Creator to help you to focus so you comprehend this important information.

All set? It's time to learn about the different types of food and the role each plays in the human body, especially as it relates to weight. We'll teach you the truth about fat, so you don't fall victim to all the confusion about fatty foods, which have the potential to cause us to gain so much weight and to put our health at risk. And remember how we promised you choices? Here is where you'll start the process of choosing how you would like to eat to lose weight. Later, in chapter 4, we'll expose you to five food pyramids, each of which offers a different way to configure your diet. You'll select the one that feels right for you and use it to guide your eating decisions. We'll also empower you to make healthy choices by teaching you how to read food labels so you can find your way through the maze of health claims.

In this chapter, we also show you that losing weight doesn't mean just eating boiled Brussels sprouts morning, noon, and night. Of course, Brussels sprouts can play a role in your healthy diet, but so can foods like chicken baked with Uncle Bubba's secret barbecue sauce, spicy seafood jambalaya, and light and fluffy coconut cream pie. While you will definitely have to exercise discipline and make some sacrifices, you won't have to feel guilty when you treat yourself. Nor will we tell you that you must eat in a way that deprives you of the wonderful sensory and spiritual pleasures that food can bring. As you read and focus during this chapter, we'll make sure that you understand that all the hard work you're going to do is well worth your effort.

So, before we teach you about food and weight loss, let's lay a good foundation. Let's first take a moment to refresh our memories—or possibly learn for the first time—about the fundamentals of good nutrition. This is the cornerstone of successful weight loss.

How to Create a Healthy Diet

Although we don't often think about food in this way, our body requires a source of energy so it can carry out essential functions—you know, eating, sleeping, shopping for shoes, watching the game. In times of plenty, we obtain this energy from food and beverages. When food is scarce, our bodies turn within, usually by burning reserves of fat. But for reasons we'll tell you about later, starving yourself—or skipping meals, in other words—can not only prevent you from losing weight, it can make it easier for you to gain. As a matter of fact—and you may be happy to learn this—*not eating* is the least effective weight-loss strategy.

We measure food energy in units called *calories*. But even though we often think about calories in a negative light, they are neither good nor bad; they're merely a unit of measure—like distance can be calculated in feet or miles, and volume in gallons or liters. Just think of it like this: Our bodies are able to obtain more energy from a food containing fifty calories than one containing twenty-five; and when we burn off two hundred calories, we expend more energy than when we burn off only one hundred. No wonder we find ourselves feeling low on energy when we skip meals or don't get enough to eat. Whether coming into our bodies or going out, calories equal energy.

Our body creates this energy from the *nutrients* it finds in our food. There are six types of nutrients: carbohydrates, fat, protein, and water—these are the *macronutrients*; and vitamins and minerals—these are the *micronutrients*. We obtain most of our energy—and, therefore, our calories—from carbohydrates, fat, and protein. However, most foods contain all six nutrients, with one or two macronutrients usually dominant. In addition to generating energy, nutrients build, maintain, and repair tissue, and carry out basic bodily functions.

Unfortunately, some people don't get enough nutrients and end up improperly nourished or even malnourished. We're not just talking about people we see on TV with bloated abdomens in developing countries; it's also possible to eat large quantities of food without getting enough—or the right kinds of—nutrition. Right here in America, where food is abundant, improper nutrition causes many common health problems, ranging from anemia to heart disease to osteoporosis. That's also how many of us become overweight—by eating a diet that is out of balance nutritionally. Let's explore the idea of nutritional balance. We'll focus on the macronutrients: carbohydrates, fat, protein, and water. As you read about them, don't worry about memorizing any numbers and percentages; just try to get a general sense of proportion. Later, we'll provide you with some handy tools that will guide your dietary decisions so you don't have to deal with any figures but your own.

Carbohydrates

These are our bodies' primary and quickest source of energy. Created through photosynthesis when plants are exposed to light, *carbohydrates* are the most abundant organic compound found in nature. Our bodies look to carbohydrates for energy before they use fat or protein. As a result, carbohydrates actually form a buffer zone that keeps our bodies from burning our own muscles (composed largely of proteins) for energy. They regulate the amount of sugar in our bloodstream, help us perform such functions as digesting food and absorbing calcium, and contain dietary fiber, another essential element of the human diet. Carbohydrates are vital, so they should comprise 60 percent of your diet. When your mama wouldn't excuse you from the dinner table until you ate your fruits and vegetables, she knew what she was doing.

Also known as "carbs," carbohydrates are categorized as either starches or sugars. Most plant-based foods are classified as *starches*, except for most fruits. So even though they look and taste dissimilar, foods like yams, rice, pasta, and black-eyed peas are all examples of starches. Fruits are classified as *sugars*—foods containing natural or added sugar. Apples, grapes, a Snickers bar, and a Pepsi all fall into the sugar category, although it probably won't surprise you to know that your body is better off when you eat fruits, which contain natural sugars, than when you indulge in snacks and beverages with added sugars. Many foods containing added sugar have been stripped of many important nutrients, including vitamins, minerals, and fiber, during the refining process.

The dietary fiber contained in unrefined carbs is important for losing weight as well as maintaining good health. Fiber helps you feel full. That's why eating a bowl of oatmeal for breakfast keeps you from getting hungry. So increasing the amount of fiber in your diet is a good weight-loss strategy. Fiber also "keeps you regular." If you've ever found yourself needing to move your bowels within a couple hours of eating a big plate of collards or gorging yourself with watermelon, fiber is the reason why. It prevents problems like constipation and hemorrhoids, and may even reduce your risk of bowel cancer, precisely because of its role in the process of elimination. Fiber also helps lower cholesterol and blood sugar, seems to offer protection against heart disease, and reduces your risk of diabetes. On the flip side, if you don't get enough fiber—and especially if you eat a lot of foods that are high in fat—you increase your risk of developing constipation, bowel cancer, or heart disease, or becoming obese. Trust us when we tell you that you're better off eating your broccoli.

But you're not likely to get much fiber if you eat a lot of processed foods. Manufacturers *refine* and *process* foods—particularly carbohydrates—to extend their shelf life and to engineer other flavors, ingredients, and characteristics into them. It's the processing that makes cereals sweet and transforms kernels of wheat into hard, dry pasta or soft, moist bread. But as we told you earlier, processing also strips food of vitamins, minerals, and dietary fiber, thereby making them less nutritious. You'll often hear processed foods referred to as "empty calories"; this means that the calories add up but don't have much nutrition in them. To get the most nutritional "bang" for every calorie you consume, we suggest you focus your diet around foods that are unrefined or that have been only lightly processed—foods like brown rice, whole-grain breads and cereals, fresh fruits and vegetables, legumes, nuts, and seeds.

The most highly processed foods—foods like white rice, white flour, white-flour pasta, and white sugar—often add up to double trouble. They tend to be not only low in nutrients, they are often ingredients in high-fat, high-calorie foods, like mass-produced baked goods, fast foods, and convenience items. They are likely to slide from your lips down to your hips, without adding much nutrition in between. The less refined the food, the better for your health, and this may require you to exercise some discipline. But it won't kill you if you throw down on a glazed doughnut from time to time. As we'll tell you later, the point is to make sure that you eat refined foods in moderation. All the more reason to enjoy your food and savor every bite as it goes down.

Fat

After carbohydrates, the body taps into fat for energy. Although many people will try to convince you that fat is the nutritional bad guy, it is actually essential to good health. *Dietary fat* (the fat found in food) is the most concentrated source of energy available to our bodies. It helps our brains develop and assists in the absorption of the fat-soluble vitamins A, D, E, and K. Fat also lends taste, texture, and aroma to foods, and, most important, leaves us feeling full. That's why some low-fat foods aren't very tasty and leave you with the sensation of wanting more. The government recommends that 30 percent of our diet come from fat—but it's important to understand what kind. Because it is the source of so much misery and confusion, we want to make sure you understand how this important nutrient works, so we'll go into more depth with this than with any of the other nutrients.

Contrary to its reputation, *body fat* is essential to good health. It gives you your shapely figure (think breasts, hips, and even your spare tire); cushions your skin and organs (imagine how painful it would be to sit on a wooden chair without the fat on your behind); insulates you from the cold (the winter is one time you want a little meat on your bones); and provides an excellent source of stored energy to protect you against starvation. So while our objective is to lose unhealthy weight, all of us need to maintain a certain amount of body fat. Actually, between 18.5 and 24 percent of your body should consist of body fat. In chapter 6 we'll help you identify where your body falls relative to this range.

What's the relationship between body fat and dietary fat? Well, people who consume a lot of dietary fat also tend to carry more body fat. That's because dietary fat has more than twice as many calories as either carbohydrates or proteins. This is important to understand, so we're going to repeat it: *Fat has more than twice as many calories per bite as carbohydrates and proteins.* One gram of fat contains 9 calories, whereas one gram of carbs or protein contains only 4 calories. So without even realizing it, people who eat a lot of foods with fat in them are likely consuming a lot more calories in the same number of bites. All the more reason not to eat a lot of high-fat foods.

But there's a second way dietary fat contributes to body fat. Whenever we eat more calories from any food source than our body needs that day, it stores the extra calories as body fat. No surprise, huh? Well, unfortunately, it gets worse. The fat in your body is very similar to the fat found in food. As a result, while your body burns calories to convert protein and carbohydrates to body fat, it hardly has to burn any when it converts dietary fat to body fat. Your body stores dietary fat pretty much "as is." (Almost 25 percent of extra carbohydrate and protein calories get burned up in the conversion to body fat versus about only 3 percent of fat calories.) When you take this conversion factor into consideration, *extra calories in the form of fat end up being about three times as fattening as extra calories from carbs or protein.*

Since many Americans eat both too many calories and too many fat calories (many of us get more than 40 percent of our calories from fat as opposed to the 30 percent maximum that the government recommends), it's no wonder that our stomachs are shaking, our booties are bouncing, and our thighs are thundering. Nor should it surprise us that we suffer so often from such fat-related dietary illnesses as heart disease, diabetes, and cancers.

Here's the bottom line: You should never attempt to eliminate fat from your diet or lose too much of it from your body. What you should do is eat the right kinds of fats and in the right amounts. But to do that, you need to understand the differences between the different types of dietary fat and the role each plays in your body. We're going to dig a little deeper into this nutrient called fat.

Dietary fat is composed of building blocks called fatty acids. There are three kinds of fatty acids—*saturated*, *polyunsaturated*, and *monounsaturated*. The differences between them boil down to how much hydrogen is in their chemical makeup. Saturated fats are literally that—saturated with hydrogen, which makes their chemical bonds extremely difficult for the body to break down and to move out of your system. Unsaturated fatty acids (whether mono- or polyunsaturated) are not loaded with hydrogen and are, therefore, easier for the body to break apart and to digest.

These three fatty acids combine to form dietary fats that bear their same names: saturated, polyunsaturated, and monounsaturated. Each type of fat actually contains all three types of fatty acids. But what type of fat a food is categorized as is determined by which fatty acid dominates.

A pork chop, which is labeled as a saturated fat, also contains monounsaturated and polyunsaturated fats (a typical pork chop is composed of 34 percent saturated fat, 16 percent polyunsaturated fat, and 16 percent monounsaturated fat). Olive oil—composed of 14 percent saturated fat, 9 percent polyunsaturated fat, and 77 percent monounsaturated fat—is categorized as a monounsaturated fat. And corn oil—13 percent saturated, 62 percent polyunsaturated fat, and 25 percent monounsaturated fat—is a polyunsaturated fat.

But here's where things can get a bit confusing: If more than one-third of the fat in a food comes from saturated fat, nutritionists label that food as a saturated fat, no matter how much of the other fatty acids are in the

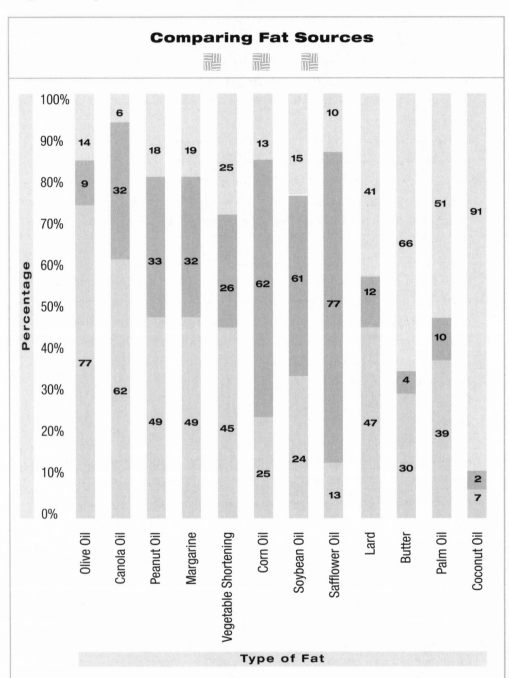

Comparing Fat Sources

Key: Top: saturated; middle: polyunsaturated; bottom: monounsaturated.

Source: Canola Council of Canada and Bertolli

food. A good example is bacon, which is labeled a saturated fat even though it contains almost equal amounts of polyunsaturated and momounsaturated fats (about 40 percent).

Saturated Fats

Like bacon, most—but not all—*saturated fats* are derived from animal products. Your body needs saturated fat, so even though you need to be careful about how much you consume, you shouldn't try to eliminate it from your diet. Still, Americans eat way too much of it, which is danger-ous because the liver uses it to manufacture cholesterol. (We'll teach you more about cholesterol shortly.) For now, just know that when you eat too much, it's akin to dialing up your liver and telling it to whip up another batch of cholesterol. High cholesterol, especially LDL cholesterol (the "bad" one), is a major risk factor for heart disease, the number one killer of African-Americans. So it's important to limit your consumption of sat-urated fats to the small amount that your body needs each day. They should comprise no more than 10 percent of your daily diet.

How do you know how to recognize saturated fats? They're usually easy to pick out because they are typically solid at room temperature (think butter, lard, and bacon grease). Foods high in saturated fats include red meats; some dairy products, like cheese, cream, and milk; and eggs. That's why nutritionists recommend you buy extra-lean meats, drink skim or 1 percent milk, consume low-fat dairy products, and eat no more than three eggs a week. Surprisingly, several vegetable products are also high in saturated fat—cocoa butter, palm oil, and coconut oil. If you cook with them, they can wreak havoc on your arteries, so best to con-sume them sparingly, if at all (better yet—save them for treating your ashy ankles).

Many people who consume too much saturated fat eat too much of the wrong types of meat. That's why your doctor will tell you to cut back on certain meats if you have high cholesterol and some other health prob-lems. The biggest culprits include bacon, ground beef, ham, lamb, lunch meats, rabbit, sausage, and steak. You should also avoid prime cuts, espe-cially when you're dining out. They usually contain a lot of saturated fat, and chefs often brush even more on to enhance the flavor. But there are some cuts of meat most of us can still enjoy without worrying about whether we're sending our cholesterol sky-high. Canadian bacon and extra-lean versions of the high-saturated-fat meats are much healthier choices, and low-fat bacon, sausage, and hot dogs can still be quite tasty. Most of the saturated fat in poultry is contained in its skin, so when you remove the skin before you cook it, you make a much healthier choice. Fish is generally great to eat because it's low in saturated fats; however, if it's processed (processed fish is usually breaded or battered, then fried), it picks up a lot of saturated fat.

Speaking of processed foods, remember how we warned you earlier to be wary of eating them? Well, in addition to being low in nutrients and high in calories, many baked goods—like pies, cookies, cakes, and pastries—are also loaded with butter and other saturated fats. And as you now know, excess fat is likely to make you gain weight. The low-fat versions of processed foods are usually healthier, especially if you don't go overboard eating them. But low-fat foods can also be dangerous. Many people gain weight because they eat a larger quantity of the low-fat version than they would if they went ahead and ate some of the full-fat food. They miss the flavor and fullness that fat provides, so they keep eating because they don't feel satisfied. What they don't realize is that they may have cut back on fat, but by eating extra servings, they may be consuming more calories than they would have had they just gone ahead and eaten the full-fat food they were trying to avoid in the first place. If you're confused by the relationship between calories and fat, you're not alone. Many of us think that because something is low in fat it's also low in calories. But calories can come from protein, carbohydrates, *or* fat and most foods contain all three, remember? A low-fat cookie can be low in fat but high in calories, so you're eating a lot of sugar. The massive confusion surrounding this issue is one reason Americans keep gaining weight despite the fact they're eating more low-fat foods.

But at the same time Americans are eating more low-fat foods, we're are also treating ourselves to more gourmet and specialty foods. Unfortunately, if you're trying to lose weight, these are the products you'll need to stay away from. The rich flavor they have often comes from added fat and much of it is saturated fat. The regular versions of ice cream and chocolate are already high in saturated fat, but the gourmet versions blow the roof off the fat count. For example, a single serving of some premium brands of ice cream contains 50 percent of the saturated fat that you should eat *in an entire day*. Low-fat ice creams are much better choices.

Okay, you've made it through the first round of nutrition information. We have a lot more we want to tell you about fat, including what kinds of fat are most healthy for you.

Unsaturated Fats

Unsaturated fats usually come from the seed or kernel of a plant. They are usually liquid at room temperature, but depending on their type, they may stay liquid or coagulate—become solid—when refrigerated. There are two types of unsaturated fats, polyunsaturated and monounsaturated.

Polyunsaturated fats stay liquid at room temperature and when refrigerated. (Think sunflower, safflower, corn, or soy oils.) There is conflicting information about whether they are good for you. At one point, scientists heralded their ability to reduce cholesterol, but now some studies suggest you should avoid them. The American Heart Association recommends you limit your intake of polyunsaturated fats to no more than 10 percent of your calories, since their long-term safety in higher amounts hasn't been proven. In any case, polyunsaturated fats certainly become much less healthy when you heat them, so if you need oil for cooking, choose one of the monounsaturated oils that are available.

Monounsaturated fats, have been found to have a positive effect on blood cholesterol—they raise levels of HDL cholesterol (the "good" one) and slightly lower levels of LDL cholesterol (the "bad" one). People whose diets are high in monounsaturated fats seem to live longer, have lower levels of obesity, and get fewer cancers than people consuming a typical American diet high in saturated fats. One of the reasons nutritionists rave about the dietary habits of people who live around the Mediterranean Sea is because of the population's reliance on monounsaturated fats and their low incidence of typical illnesses and diseases that strike Americans.

Where can you find monounsaturated fats? They're usually found in vegetable and nut oils, like canola, olive, and peanut. They are also found in olives themselves, avocados, hummus (a puree of chickpeas common to the Mediterranean and Middle East), and many types of nuts, including macadamia and hazel nuts. (Be careful: Nuts contain very high amounts of fat, and fats are high in calories, remember?) Typically liquid at room temperature, monounsaturated fats will thicken or harden when cooled. (Try refrigerating canola oil and watch what happens.) If you use oil to cook with, olive oil is healthiest. Aim to increase the amount of monounsaturated fats in your diet. If possible, use them to replace saturated or polyunsaturated fats.

The Dangers of Trans-fats

Trans-fats are another important category of fat you need to be aware of, primarily because they contribute to high cholesterol. They are man-made fats, created when unsaturated oils, like corn and soybean, are processed by adding more hydrogen to them. This process, referred to as *hydrogenation* (you may see trans-fats referred to on food labels as "partially hydrogenated fats"), makes oils hard at room temperature. The extra hydrogen *trans*forms the easily digestible unsaturated fats into a saturated fat, which is much more difficult for your body to break down. Stick margarines are a common example. Other trans-fats are created for commercial baking and frying.

But in spite of the convenience they may bring, there's a tremendous problem with trans-fats. Recent studies show that they not only reduce HDL cholesterol levels, but they raise LDL cholesterol levels. So try to steer clear of any label containing the words "hydrogenated" or "partially hydrogenated fat." If you must consume trans-fats regularly, choose ones where the partially hydrogenated item appears as the second ingredient on the food label.

 Nutritional Fish Stories

Over the past recent years, the health benefits of Omega-3 fatty acids have been splashed all over the media. Omega-3 fats are unsaturated oils that are primarily found in fatty fish, such as Atlantic and coho salmon, albacore tuna, club mackerel, carp, lake whitefish, sweet smelt, and lake and brook trout.

Currently the subject of much investigation, Omega-3 oils may help keep bones from breaking down and even help build new bone; they may relieve the pain, inflammation, and swelling caused by arthritis; seem to have cholesterol-lowering benefits; and help regulate the moods of people who suffer from bipo-lar disorder (also known as manic depression).

No word yet on how much Omega-3s you should consume each day, but many experts recommend that we increase our consumption of fish to two or more servings a week.

Cholesterol

Just as your body needs all types of fat, it needs *cholesterol*, as well. For all the negative press it receives, cholesterol is a vital part of the structure of your cells. It helps your nerves send and receive information, assists you in absorbing fats and fat-soluble vitamins, and is used to manufacture sex hormones. If it weren't for cholesterol, you wouldn't be able to "get it on"—nor would people be able to get on your nerves.

Cholesterol enters your bloodstream through two sources: your liver manufactures it (*serum cholesterol*) and you consume it in food (*dietary cholesterol*). If everything's in balance and functioning as it should, the HDL ("good") cholesterol carries any excess cholesterol that happens to be hanging around, out of your bloodstream and into the liver, where it's broken down for excretion from the body. But if there's too much choles-terol in your system, your HDLs become outnumbered and can't elimi-nate cholesterol quickly enough. The excess cholesterol forms a plaque that sticks to artery walls and may eventually cause heart attack or stroke.

This is why it's so important to be careful about the amount of satu-rated fat you eat. Remember, one of the roles of saturated fat is to tell your body to produce serum cholesterol. And excess saturated fat will sig-nal to your body that it should produce extra cholesterol. Know, too, that not only do foods of animal origin contain saturated fat, they are also one of the primary sources of dietary cholesterol. (Plant-based foods, like nuts, can be high in fat, but no food from a plant contains cholesterol.) So try to moderate your consumption of meat and limit organ meats such as brains, hearts, kidneys, liver, and sweetbreads, which contain very high amounts of cholesterol. And as we told you earlier, be aware of the amount of full-fat dairy products you eat, especially butter, cream, and ice cream; and try to limit yourself to three egg yolks per week.

So while we try to keep you from having to remember a lot of numbers, your dietary cholesterol is one to keep an eye on—particularly if you are predisposed to heart disease. Limit your intake of dietary cholesterol to 300 or fewer milligrams per day.

Protein

Protein is the third type of food the body uses to perform its daily functions. The body uses protein to make and repair cells (especially muscles) and to generate new proteins that help it perform its basic bodily functions. If you don't get enough protein in your diet, your body will digest the protein in your body, including muscle tissue. This is why starving people look like they are composed of skin and bones—they literally are.

Protein, like fats, are composed of building blocks. The building blocks of protein are called *amino acids* and are found in both plant and animal foods. Because people and animals are both—well, animals—the combinations of amino acids found in animal products, like meat, poultry, fish, eggs, and dairy products, are most similar to those found in the human body. As a result, animal protein is referred to as a "complete protein." Vegetable protein is termed "incomplete" because it's missing certain amino acids.

Only about 10 percent of our diet should consist of protein—a guideline that is especially important to adhere to since most animal products contain saturated fats *and* cholesterol, both of which we're trying to minimize in our diets. Not surprisingly, most Americans eat way too much animal protein. Diets that are too high in protein, particularly animal protein (and including high-protein weight-loss diets) have been linked to bone demineralization, osteoporosis, and kidney stones. They may also have a negative effect on kidney function.

So what are good—and healthy—sources of protein? Egg whites are one of the best sources (the yolks are high in cholesterol), so experiment with an egg-white omelet one day. Poultry and fish—especially fish—are great protein sources with reasonable levels of saturated fat and cholesterol.

Vegetable protein can be found in legumes, grains, nuts, and seeds. The best source of vegetable protein is the wonderful soybean, which is the only plant food that contains all of the amino acids available in meat. The best thing about the soybean is that it contains none of the cholesterol and little saturated fat (it can be high in unsaturated fat, though, so look for low-fat versions). This is one of many reasons tofu and other soy-based foods, like soy milk, soy burgers, and other "fake" meats, have become so popular in recent years.

If you're a vegetarian or don't eat much meat, try to incorporate soy into your diet. In addition to soy, the best way to get enough protein is to eat several different kinds of vegetable protein at some point during the day. That's one of many reasons it's very important for vegetarians to eat a wide variety of carbohydrates rather than relying on the same old, same old, day after day.

Contrary to popular belief, you don't have to combine vegetable proteins into one dish or even one meal; you just need to make sure to eat them at some time during the day. Having said that, however, it's easier to combine veggie proteins in the same dish or meal, just so you don't forget later. (We'll teach you more about the food combining in the next chapter, in the section covering the Vegetarian Pyramid. It's an amazing science that's as old—and intuitive—as the stars.)

 What's a Legume?

If you've gotta say it in French, it must be too high-falutin' for me, you may be thinking. But you probably eat legumes all the time.

Pronounced lay-GOOM, these are merely unshelled beans or peas—the beans or peas that are still in the pod. Think green beans or snap beans; they're legumes. We're accustomed to eating both the bean and the pod, but if we were to split it open, we'd be eating the peas alone. Other examples of legumes are chickpeas (also known as garbanzo beans) and lentils.

Water

No conversation about nutrition is complete without at least a brief discussion of water. The human body is composed of about two-thirds water. Water helps you digest food, carries nutrients through your system and waste out of your body, facilitates your metabolic processes, regulates your body temperature, and lubricates all your moving parts. Without it, you won't get very far.

Water is so important that your body has a miraculous mechanism to let you know when you need more—you get thirsty. Thirst is your body's way of reminding you to bring your water content back in balance. If you ignore your thirst—or take diet pills or employ weight-loss strategies that cause you to lose water weight—your body will go through a series of increasingly severe stages of dehydration. First, you'll lose your appetite. At first, you may interpret that as a good thing, but before long, you'll start to feel "off," as water is drained from your blood cells and deployed to other areas of your body. Next you'll feel tired, nauseated, get a headache, and even become flushed. Soon, your body will begin to shut down and you'll require hospitalization.

Water is an important element of any weight-loss strategy. If you don't drink enough of it, your body desperately hangs on to what little it has, creating what we know as *water weight*. So contrary to popular belief, water weight is not eliminated by drinking less water. Not only will drinking enough water keep you from being bloated, it will help you feel full and energetic, and help your body to move waste out of your system. You should drink at least 64 ounces of water a day, especially when you're losing weight. That's eight 8-ounce glasses, two liters of bottled water, or a gallon jug of water. *Every day!* You'll need more to offset your perspiration when you start the exercise portion of your *HealthQuest* 30-Day Weight-Loss Program.

Sodium

No conversation about weight-loss, water, or Black health is complete without a mention of sodium. Sodium is a type of mineral called an *electrolyte*. It helps the body maintain the proper balance of fluid outside and inside each cell. When sodium is in the proper balance, our cells don't dry up and die nor do they fill up and explode. It also plays a vital role in stomach, nerve, and muscle function.

Most of us are familiar with sodium in the form of table salt (sodium chloride), but it also occurs naturally in virtually all foods. Most Americans—especially African-Americans—consume way too much sodium. "We're eating at least eight times more than other [races]," says nutritionist Dr. Goulda Downer. Eating too much sodium increases the risk of high blood pressure and heart disease among those of us whose systems are sensitive to sodium. No wonder hypertension runs rampant in our community.

What's the relationship between sodium and heart disease? Sodium attracts and holds on to water. When you eat too much sodium, too much water floods your vascular system, and your heart is forced to work overtime to pump it out. Eventually your heart wears down and is unable to clear all the fluid. That's why sufferers of heart disease begin to retain fluid in their legs, become short of breath (your lungs begin to fill with fluid), and have a hard time lying down. Recently scientists have discovered a specific "salt" gene, which may explain why some people can reduce their blood pressure by cutting back on salt, while others aren't affected by salt at all. More research on the salt gene needs to be done before we understand its health implications.

Reducing salt also has an important weight-loss benefit. If you eat less salt, your body won't hold on to excess water. It will use water and move it out of your system, instead. You won't feel bloated and you'll look and feel thinner.

The government recommends that we consume no more than 2,400 milligrams of sodium daily. That's the equivalent of a level teaspoon of salt. But remember: Sodium occurs naturally in many foods and is added to others, so most of us can leave the salt shaker off the table. Here are some additional ways you can avoid getting too much sodium:

• *Read food labels.* Look for items with less than 400 milligrams of sodium per serving. But you have to read carefully. Some foods labeled "reduced sodium" may still be a significant source of sodium, especially canned soups, chicken broth, and soy sauce. And even foods that aren't salty, like cookies, candy, and sodas, can be high in sodium.

• *Limit processed foods.* Canned foods, processed meats, and some frozen meals (even vegetables in sauce) are often heavily salted.

• *Limit high-salt snacks.* Go for unsalted crackers, pretzels, and chips.

• *Watch your medications.* Aspirin, cold medicines, cough medicine, and laxatives may be high in sodium, according to Dr. Downer.

• *Season carefully.* Baking powder, baking soda, and bouillon are salty, as are mixed spices like garlic salt, seasoning salt, and even some brands of lemon pepper. Use herbs and spices instead.

• *Stay off the spreads and sauces.* Ketchup, mustard, barbecue sauce, and other condiments are loaded with salt.

How to Read Food Labels

Any conversation about nutrition begs the question of food labels and how to read them. To help you sort through the nutritional maze, the government requires that consumer-friendly labels appear on almost all food packaging (the exception being items like chewing gum, spices, coffee, and bakery items, which contain minimal amounts of nutrients or whose nutrient content varies from batch to batch). The labels, entitled "Nutritional Facts," must include certain nutritional information, accurate ingredient listings, and reliable information about whether a food is high or low in nutrients.

1. **Serving size.** This part of the label makes serving sizes understandable, translating them from grams and other difficult quantities into real-world measurements like cups and slices. To make nutritional comparisons easier, items within the same food category must depict the same serving size. For instance, all soups must use the same serving size so you can compare them to each other.

   But here's the tricky part: Always look at the serving size carefully. Not only do serving sizes on food labels not correspond to serving sizes recommended in the Food Guide Pyramid, they may not even reflect the amount a typical adult may eat. For instance, the serving size for potato chips may be one ounce, but many bags you'll find at the lunch counter at your favorite deli contain two ounces or more. Besides, when was the last time you threw down on just a couple of chips?

Nutrition Facts

1

Serving Size: 1 cup (238 g)
Servings per container: 2

2

Amount per Serving

Calories 90   Calories from fat 10

3

	% Daily Value*
Total Fat 2g	3%
Saturated Fat 0g	0%
Cholesterol 10mg	3%
Sodium 890mg	37%
Total Carbohydrate 13g	4%
Dietary Fiber 1g	4%
Sugars 1g	
Protein 6g	

Vitamin A 20%	Vitamin C 0%
Calcium 0%	Iron 2%

4

*Percent Daily Values are based on a 2,000-calorie diet. Your daily values may be higher or lower depending on your calorie needs.

	Calories	2,000	2,500
Total Fat	Less than	65g	80g
Sat. Fat	Less than	20g	25g
Cholesterol	Less than	300mg	300mg
Sodium	Less than	2,400mg	2,400mg
Total carbohydrate		300g	375mg
Dietary fiber		25g	30g

2. **Calories.** This figure is more straightforward. It provides the number of calories contained in a single serving, whatever size that serving is. Also look for "Calories from Fat"—the actual number of calories that come from fat—the lower the percentage of the total number of calories, the better.

3. **Percent Daily Values.** This portion of the label shows whether a food is high or low in a particular nutrient. It depicts the percentage of nutrients one serving contributes to a 2,000-calorie daily diet. But this is another place to be careful, especially if you're on a diet. Many women and children should eat less than 2,000 calories per day. As a rule of thumb, consider a daily value of 5 percent or less to be low in a nutrient and 20 percent or more as high.

4. **Footnote.** Here are the nutritional values of the most important vitamins and nutrients in the product, although not all of them.

Evaluating Health Claims

There's another important aspect of reading food labels. To get the full effect, try walking down the cereal aisle. You'll be amazed how many breakfast foods, particularly those marketed to adults (the ones at an adult's-eye level), claim to work health magic. Forget the wonders of herbal remedies or pharmaceutical drugs, you'd think you could be cured of everything that ails you just by eating cereal. But what does this information mean? And, more important, can you trust it?

The government allows manufacturers to make health claims based only upon well-documented scientific studies that have proven the relationship between the following factors:

- calcium and bone density
- a high-fat diet and a higher risk of cancer
- a diet high in fat, saturated fat, and cholesterol and a higher risk of heart disease
- a higher-fiber diet and a lower risk of some kinds of cancer
- a high-fiber diet and a lower risk of heart attack
- sodium and hypertension (high blood pressure)
- a diet rich in fruits and vegetables and a low risk of some types of cancer

For instance, a label may legitimately read: "High in calcium," "This food follows the recommendations of the American Heart Association's diet to lower the risk of heart disease," or "Foods high in dietary fiber may help reduce the risk of coronary heart disease."

But how high is high and how low is low? For that, you have to turn to a different set of definitions. If you see the following terms on a food label, they conform to these strict definitions:

- *Lite (or Light)* can be used to describe the calorie, fat, or sodium content of a food, although the definition of a food labeled light in calories is different than the definition for foods light in fat and sodium. A food that contains one-third the amount of calories of the comparable product can be labeled "light," as can products containing 50 percent less fat or 50 percent less sodium. (For instance, lite wheat bread must have no more than one-third the amount of calories of regular wheat bread.)

- *Reduced Sodium* means a product contains at least 25 percent less sodium than the original product.

- *Low Sodium* means a product contains less than 140 milligrams of sodium per serving. (For the average person, no more than 2,400 milligrams of sodium per day are advised.)

- *Sodium-Free* means less than 5 milligrams of sodium per serving. (When used on a label, the word "free" means that a food has a negligible amount, not none.)

- *Fat-Free* products must contain less than half of 1 percent of fat in a single serving.

- *Reduced Fat* means a product contains at least 25 percent less fat than the original product.

- *Low Fat* means that a food has 3 grams of fat or less per serving. (According to the FDA, 65 to 80 grams of fat per day should be the limit for the average person.)

- *Low Saturated Fat* means that a food has one gram or less of saturated fat. (According to the FDA, less than 10 percent of daily calories should come from saturated fat.)

- *Low Calorie* means a product has less than 40 calories per serving. (For the average person, 2,000 to 2,500 calories per day are recommended.)

- *Low Cholesterol* products contain 20 milligrams or less of cholesterol per serving. (The FDA says the average person should have no more than 300 milligrams of cholesterol daily.)

- *Cholesterol-Free* means less than 2 milligrams of cholesterol or 2 grams or less of saturated fat.

Think It Through

L ook at your Food and Fitness Diary entries for the entire week, paying special attention to your comments on how you were feeling when you ate a given food. Do you find any patterns? Look for things like eating to be sociable, eating when you're angry or lonely, eating to reward yourself.

Now, think of how you might have handled the emotions you were feeling in some other way besides eating. Create a substitutions list. List all of the occasions when you might overeat for emotional or social reasons. Then make a list of things you can do instead of eating. (Try to cover not only the scenarios from your week-long food diary, but other situations that come up often.) Pick a food substitute that fits your circumstances and personality. And choose things that match the emotion you're feeling. If you're agitated, it helps to do something active to get your mind off of it. Or if you're feeling lonely, you'll want to do something that gives you human contact. Your list might look something like this:

> *Stressed at work:* Get out of the office and walk around the block. Stop working straight through lunch. Come home and work on my hobby (knitting, woodworking, etc.), play cards, work a puzzle.
> *Lonely:* Call a friend on the phone or go visit a neighbor. Write some letters. Take a class. Schedule some volunteer work.
> *Mad at the kids:* Write about it in my journal. Put on some funky music and dance.
> *Needing a reward:* Go buy a new CD or book. Treat myself to a video or go to a movie.
> *Bored:* Cruise the Internet. Read. Go for a walk.

For Your Spirit

Trying to keep up in this fast-paced world can cause us to miss a lot of joy. The joy of eating is a prime example. Eating is a fundamental human need, something we all have to do to live. And you can get nourishment from your food without enjoying it. But why would you—especially when you're trying to lose weight? As Black folks in America, we have more than our share of unpleasantness to cope with. Eating a delicious, healthy meal can be one moment in your day that you savor and enjoy.

Practice eating with awareness—slowing down enough to really pay attention to what you're cooking and eating.

Before nourishment passes by your lips—whether it's juice and a bagel in the morning or Sunday dinner with all the trimmings—close your eyes and pause to give thanks. When you open your eyes, notice the colors before you. Are they pale and gentle, or intense and vibrant? Do the colors of the meal come from the same family, like the yellows, browns, and reds of a cornbread and chili dinner, or are they a lovely mélange, like fruit salad?

Bring the first forkful of each food to your nostrils and inhale. Warm foods have aromas, but even cold foods—like potato salad or vanilla ice cream—do, too. It's just that we usually don't take the time to appreciate them. As you open your mouth, keep opening your senses. Hear the juicy crunch of an ear of corn on the cob. Listen for the sound that a pear makes when you bite into it.

Pay attention to how the food feels in your mouth. What kind of textures are rolling on your tongue? Delight in the smoothness of a banana, the creaminess of a new potato.

And finally, pay attention to taste—the pleasant bitterness of turnip greens, the sweet warmth of a baked apple, the salty bite of a dill pickle.

Now take a moment to write about food. Are there certain foods and flavors you prefer more than others? If so, explore them on paper. Some of us can't wait for summer to come because we love eating fresh fruit. We love to shop for it, carve into its juicy pulp, bite into its rich red, pink, or golden flesh and wipe the juice that escapes the corners of our mouths.

Others love fresh vegetables. They love going to the farmer's market on Saturday morning, inspecting the produce to make sure it's fresh, and carrying it home to cook. Maybe you're lucky enough to have your own vegetable garden or plants you grow on your roof or fire escape. Perhaps you enjoy the scent and smell of the soil, turning over the dark earth, placing seeds or seedlings into the ground and watching them grow. Even if your garden is in your kitchen, you love keeping an eye on your hot chili peppers as they ripen or the fragrance of fresh basil as it sprawls akimbo across the windowsill.

Now get to the part where you write about eating. Perhaps you're the type of person who puts hot sauce on everything. You enjoy chowing down on spicy foods, love the tingle you get on your tongue, the way your sinuses clear, sweat beads on your forehead, and your eyes water. If so, write about it. Or maybe you jones for the flavorful seasonings of Caribbean food—zesty lime juice, fresh cilantro, sweet coconut milk, and a dash of pimento. Whatever your pleasure, put it on paper. Maybe for you food is a great prelude to sex. You enjoy eating oysters, chocolate, and other foods reputed to be aphrodisiacs. You eat at a table for two after sundown and always light a candle. If so, why not write about that? Or perhaps you have a sweet tooth that's irresistible. Whenever you go out to eat, you don't order your entrée until you see what's for dessert. Whatever your food preference, explore it on paper—and write about it with passion. Write about flavors, textures, aromas, colors, and foods you love to eat. And bring that awareness with you when you sit down to the table.

When you are eating with awareness—eating mindfully—you're more likely to really taste and enjoy your food. This is especially significant when you're on a diet—but is important any time—because you want your meals to be filling not only to your body, but to your soul and spirit as well.

Practice eating mindfully. Before long, you may find it's a pleasant habit.

CHAPTER 4

Determining Your Structure

The Food Guide Pyramids

Now that you know more about the nutrients our bodies need, you can see how important it is to eat the right foods in the right proportions if you're going to lose weight and become healthier. But the government's dietary guidelines in numbers, milligrams, and percentages still leave us with a problem: We don't know about your friends, but no one we know is going to walk around tracking their daily nutrient count, and you darn sure can't eat percentages. There's gotta be a better way, right?

Well, there is. We suggest you follow the guidance of a food pyramid, so in this chapter we'll present you with five: the USDA's Food Guide Pyramid, which is the basis for all other food pyramids; the *HealthQuest* Soul Food Pyramid; the Ethnic Food Pyramid; the Vegetarian Food Pyramid; and the Diabetes Soul Food Pyramid.

What is a food pyramid? you may ask. A food pyramid is a visual representation of the components of a healthy diet. Since no one can possibly keep track of the number of milligrams of micronutrients—the vitamins and minerals in your diet—they consume each day, you can just follow the proportions suggested in the food pyramid, and you'll get the nutrition you need.

The pyramid shape reflects the importance of balance. A balanced diet contains some foods you should eat more of and others you should eat less of. Foods depicted at the base of the pyramid form the foundation of your diet, so you eat them at every meal. The foods at the top should be eaten infrequently or in small amounts; the ones in the middle, several times a day. You'll eat a lovin' spoonful of this and a pinch of that (we'll tell you more about the number of servings and serving sizes later in the chapter), and you can enjoy everything you eat without feeling guilty.

Why do I need five food pyramids? Actually, you don't; you only need the one that's right for you. For reasons we'll explain shortly, we give you a choice between the recommendations the government makes for all Americans and the recommendations that have been developed especially for people of color (remember, we have a different ancestral diet and health issues than people of European descent). If you're a vegetarian, or aspire to be one, you can follow the veggie pyramid; if you're not, don't. It's that simple.

The USDA Food Guide Pyramid

You've probably seen the USDA Food Guide Pyramid in pamphlets in your doctor's office or on cereal boxes or bread wrappers. It depicts the government's official recommendations on healthy eating. Let's take a closer look at it.

The wide base of the Food Guide Pyramid is composed of grains—breads, cereals, rice, and pasta. These foods should form the foundation of your diet. Eat more servings of grains each day than of any other type of food.

Move up the pyramid one level and you'll find fruits and vegetables. You should eat a number of fruits and vegetables each day, but not as many servings as grain-based foods. Consistent with the fact that carbohydrates form the basis of the human diet, these three bottom layers of the pyramid—the grain layer and the fruits and veggies layers—are composed of plant-based foods, the carbs your body needs for energy.

Now move to the third level of the pyramid, where you'll find the milk, yogurt, and cheese group, alongside the meat, poultry, fish, dried beans, eggs, and nuts group. These two groups of food supply you with calcium, protein, and fats. You'll eat fewer servings of these foods than of foods from the carbohydrate groups. Finally, at the top of the pyramid, you'll find foods you should eat only occasionally and in small amounts, like cooking fats, oils, and sweets.

This guidance leaves you with the obvious question of how much of each type of food you should eat, right? Well, the government's direction

USDA Food Guide Pyramid

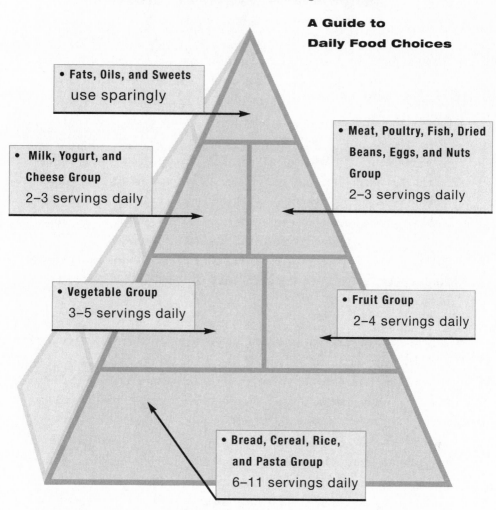

A Guide to Daily Food Choices

• Fats, Oils, and Sweets
use sparingly

• Milk, Yogurt, and Cheese Group
2–3 servings daily

• Meat, Poultry, Fish, Dried Beans, Eggs, and Nuts Group
2–3 servings daily

• Vegetable Group
3–5 servings daily

• Fruit Group
2–4 servings daily

• Bread, Cereal, Rice, and Pasta Group
6–11 servings daily

Source: U.S. Department of Agriculture/U.S. Department of Health and Human Services

follows—but don't get intimidated (or carried away) by the high number of servings you're supposed to eat; we don't want to scare you into thinking you're going to gain weight, not lose it. For now, just take note of the types of foods you should start to eat more or less of and the type of nutrition each provides. Later in the chapter we'll explain more about serving sizes. (Trust us when we tell you that healthy serving sizes are not as large as you'd think. . . .)

- **Breads, cereals, rice, and pasta—6 to 11 servings.** This is the grain group, and these foods contribute energy-storing carbohydrates and fiber. Grains also provide significant amounts of protein, B vitamins, and iron. Try eating more brown rice, bulgur (cracked wheat), kasha (buckwheat groats), graham flour, oatmeal, cornmeal, popcorn, tabouli, couscous (semolina), and whole grains like whole oats, whole rye, and whole wheat. (Note that enriched flour and wheat flour are refined, processed foods and are not considered whole grains.)

- **Vegetables—3 to 5 servings.** Vegetables also provide the body the carbohydrates needed for energy, but they also supply an array of vitamins and minerals, along with much-needed fiber and water. You should eat a wide variety of vegetables, to ensure you get the nutrients you need. Enjoy dark, leafy green vegetables, like spinach, collards, and kale; vibrant colored vegetables, like carrots, sweet potatoes, squashes, and colored peppers; and fibrous vegetables, such as broccoli, cabbage, and cauliflower.

- **Fruits—2 to 4 servings.** Fruits, like vegetables, are a vital source of carbohydrates, vitamins (especially A and C), minerals (like potassium, which helps control hypertension by flushing sodium out of your body), fiber, and water. The added bonus is that they supply the body with natural sugar—they're sweet and they taste good. Indulge in the fruits you love, whether it's citrus fruits, like oranges, grapefruits, and tangerines; firm, fibrous, crunchy fruits, like apples and pears; melons, such as watermelon, honeydew, and cantaloupe; or the "exotics," kiwi, persimmon, papaya, cherimoya, and pomegranate, to name but a few. And don't forget nature's own sweet-nibblers—berries! Strawberries, blueberries, raspberries, blackberries—all are an excellent, nutritious, fibrous snack that needs little preparation and goes a long way in providing satisfaction.

- **Milk, yogurt, and cheese—2 to 3 servings (3 servings for teens).** Dairy products contribute calcium, protein, vitamin D, and riboflavin (vitamin B$_2$). Look for nonfat (skim) and low-fat (1 percent fat) varieties of milks, yogurts, cheeses, and puddings and dairy shakes. Look for the newer vitamin D– and calcium-fortified skim milks, which are creamier and better tasting than other nonfat milks. And many nonfat and low-fat cheeses are just as delicious and melt as gloriously as their full-fat counterparts. Try nonfat yogurts sweetened with aspartame, for a good source of calcium with limited calories; or, better even, nonfat plain yogurt with some fresh pineapple.

• **Meat, poultry, fish, dried beans, eggs, and nuts—2 to 3 servings.** These foods provide the body's protein requirements, along with the B vitamins thiamin (B_1) and riboflavin (B_2), niacin, iron, and zinc. Look for extra-lean selections when buying meats (beef, ham, lamb, veal, pork) and trim off any visible fat. Chicken and turkey are the better choice when looking for a good, low-fat protein source, and fish can't be beat when it comes to protein power, essential "good fat" oils, and ease and variety in selection and preparation. Beans and legumes are an excellent, fiber-packed protein source that come in a variety of flavors, colors, shapes, and textures—explore these, by all means. Eggs, though we recommend limiting to no more than three egg yolks a week, can be enhanced by using egg whites and egg substitutes. Nuts are tasty, but remember: They are high in fat, so, unless you are a vegetarian, approach these with some caution. (Read the food label on a small bag of salted peanuts and you'll understand where we're coming from with this advice.)

• **Fats, oils, and sweets—USE SPARINGLY.** This group includes butter, margarine, mayonnaise, salad dressing, sour cream, cream cheese, potato chips, candy, cookies, cakes, pies, jams, jellies, soft drinks, fruit drinks, sherbet, and most other things shiny, oily, greasy, or sweet. Eat these foods as infrequently as possible—but enjoy them when you eat them.

If you eat the lower number of servings and adhere to the recommended serving sizes, you'll consume about 1,600 calories per day, a healthy amount for most women who don't exercise, are older, or are trying to lose weight. Consume the number of servings in the middle of the range, and you'll get around 2,200 calories, enough for most children, active women who want to maintain their weight, and sedentary men. If you consume the maximum number of servings for each food group, you'll consume about 2,800 calories daily, the amount needed by teenage boys, active men, and some extremely active women. So, again, don't be intimidated by the number of servings. Later in this chapter we'll explain serving sizes (see "Size Does Matter," on page 72) and how you can easily eat that many servings without gaining weight or feeling stuffed.

The *HealthQuest* Soul Food Pyramid

If the foods in the government Food Guide Pyramid don't appeal to you, don't feel discouraged; we've got you covered. We're going to hip you to a food pyramid with soul.

The *HealthQuest* Soul Food Pyramid, created by dietitian Constance Brown-Riggs, takes the Food Guide Pyramid and fills it with soul food. The advice and proportions are basically the same, with the top tier divided in two, but this version will help you relate our cultural foods to the proper categories on the pyramid. So if you don't know what tabouli is, there's no need to worry; we know you're familiar with cornbread. And if spinach isn't your thing, we know you'll know what to do with some collards.

So you can get a sense of how the Food Guide Pyramid can be adapted to fit Black soul food dietary practices, here are some soul foods broken out into their pyramid tiers, along with the recommended serving sizes:

- **Fats and oils—SPARINGLY**
    1 teaspoon lard
    1 slice bacon
    ¼ ounce fatback
    1 ounce hog jowls, chitterlings, or cracklin'
    1 ounce red-eye gravy

- **Sweets, salty snacks, alcohol, soda—SPARINGLY**
    ½ cup cobbler
    1 slice pound cake
    1 cup sweet tea or lemonade

HealthQuest Soul Food Pyramid

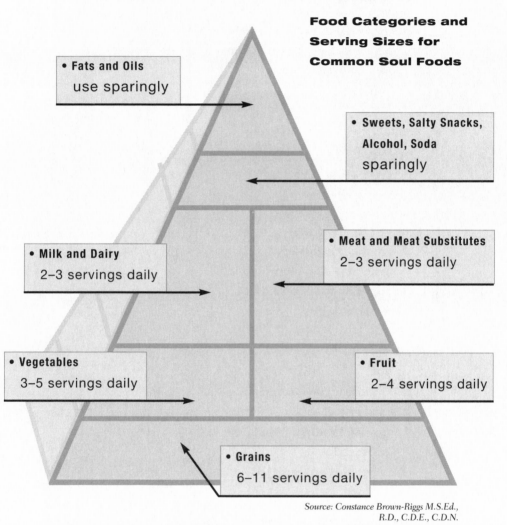

Food Categories and Serving Sizes for Common Soul Foods

- **Fats and Oils**
  use sparingly

- **Sweets, Salty Snacks, Alcohol, Soda**
  sparingly

- **Milk and Dairy**
  2–3 servings daily

- **Meat and Meat Substitutes**
  2–3 servings daily

- **Vegetables**
  3–5 servings daily

- **Fruit**
  2–4 servings daily

- **Grains**
  6–11 servings daily

Source: Constance Brown-Riggs M.S.Ed.,
R.D., C.D.E., C.D.N.

¼ cup salted nuts, chips
1 cup soda
1 ounce alcohol

- **Milk and dairy—2 to 3 servings**
  1 cup lowfat buttermilk
  ½ cup evaporated skim milk
  ½ cup ice cream or frozen yogurt
  1½ ounces Cheddar cheese

- **Meat and meat substitutes—2 to 3 servings**

  1 egg

  $\frac{1}{2}$ cup cooked black-eyed peas or lima beans

  2 to 3 ounces cooked neck bones, pig's feet, hog jowls,
  catfish, trout

  $\frac{1}{3}$ cup nuts

- **Vegetables—3 to 5 servings**

  $\frac{1}{2}$ cup cooked kale, collard greens, dandelion greens,
  cabbage, turnips

  $\frac{3}{4}$ cup vegetable juice

- **Fruit—2 to 4 servings**

  1 cup watermelon

  1 medium peach, plum, or apple

  $\frac{1}{2}$ cup canned or cooked fruit

  $\frac{3}{4}$ cup fruit juice

- **Grains—6 to 11 servings**

  $\frac{1}{2}$ cup cooked hominy grits, cereal, rice, or pasta

  1 ounce ready-to-eat cereal

  1 small biscuit, roll, or muffin

  $\frac{1}{2}$ English muffin or hamburger bun

  1 slice bread

  2-inch-cube cornbread

The Ethnic Food Pyramid

Some health- and civil-rights advocates criticize the dietary guidelines provided by the federal government, including many people and organizations we trust, like former U.S. Surgeon General Joycelyn Elders, M.D.; U.S. Representative Jesse Jackson Jr.; Martin Luther King III; Muhammad Ali; the Congressional Black Caucus; the NAACP; and the National Black Nurses Association. Many of these activists believe that the government's guidelines constitute a one-size-fits-all approach that's fine for people of European descent but is inappropriate for African-

Americans and other people of color. They, along with leaders from the Asian-, Hispanic-, and Native American communities, are working to influence the government to revise its standards.

What's the problem? you ask. We live in an increasingly diversifying nation. People whose ancestry is non-European have different dietary needs than people of European descent. Blacks, Latinos, Native Americans, and some Asians also tend to experience diet-related health conditions at rates higher than the general population. As a result, some civil-rights leaders and health advocates have gone so far as to claim that the government's dietary guidelines are good only for healthy folks, but the same guidelines promote disease among others. Most of their complaints have to do with the prominent position meat and dairy products have in the pyramid.

One literal bone of contention is the recommendation that Americans consume 2 to 3 servings from the milk group daily, so that they get enough calcium to prevent osteoporosis. After childhood, about 70 percent of African-Americans (and most other people who are not of northern European descent) become lactose intolerant and are, therefore, unable to digest dairy products without experiencing abdominal discomfort in the form of gas, bloating, cramping, and/or diarrhea. Not surprisingly, these people shy away from dairy products. Knowing this, the U.S. Department of Agriculture still instructs Americans to consume 2 to 3 servings of dairy products a day. Dairy products are not the only good source of calcium. Some soul food staples, like collard greens, kale, and other dark green, leafy vegetables, are also good sources, but these are de-emphasized in favor of dairy products.

Now, in the interest of fairness, we should note that the government's backers contend that lactose intolerance is a much less important problem than calcium deficiency, that indigestion is much less a problem than broken bones. They say most people who are lactose intolerant experience only mild symptoms, that dairy is a much more concentrated source of calcium than leafy green vegetables and one that more people are likely to embrace. They suggest that lactose-free products are good high-calcium alternatives, as are yogurts and certain cheeses.

But the government's critics are very adamant. "The U.S. Dietary Guidelines ignore the needs and health of minority Americans," says

Milton R. Mills, M.D., a medical director and critical-care physician in northern Virginia and associate director of preventive medicine for the Physicans Committee for Responsible Medicine (PCRM), one of the government's most vocal critics. "Studies show that minorities have higher rates of diabetes, prostate cancer, and other diseases than Whites, but federal food policy still pushes milk and meat, which aggravate these epidemics."

A study entitled "Racial Bias in Federal Nutrition Policy," performed by Dr. Mills and several colleagues and published in the *Journal of the National Medical Association*, concludes that federal guidelines "may encourage a disproportionate toll or chronic disease among minorities." The civil-rights leaders and health advocates listed above all agree, and a lawsuit has been filed against the government for promoting the current guidelines.

It's up to you to decide whom to believe. Perhaps you'd like to do your own investigation. In any case, we'd like you to take a look at the Ethnic Food Pyramid, created by nutritionist Dr. Goulda Downer. It contains dietary guidance relevant to people who are not of northern European descent.

The Ethnic Food Pyramid works the same way as the USDA Food Guide Pyramid; you eat more of the foods located at the bottom of the Pyramid and fewer servings of the foods located at the top. But it compensates for the fact that most people of color are lactose intolerant and, as a result, need alternative sources of calcium. Notice that dairy products are "demoted" to the top of the pyramid with fats, sweets, and other foods you should eat only occasionally and in small quantities. To help ensure that you get your calcium and carbohydrates, leafy green vegetables and fruits have been "promoted" to the base of the pyramid, along with the grain group. (Dr. Downer also recommends that we consume calcium-fortified 100 percent orange juice.) That means you get to enjoy more cultural favorites like callaloo, collard greens, sweet potatoes, rice and peas, and Hoppin' John.

You'll also notice that the guidelines for the Ethnic Food Pyramid are more general than the guidelines from the Food Guide Pyramid. You're directed to "Enjoy daily at most meals," "Enjoy daily," or "Enjoy occasionally in small quantities," rather than to count servings. You'll notice

Ethnic Food Pyramid

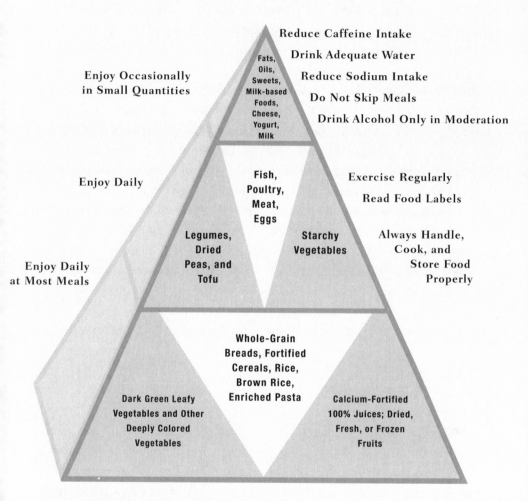

Reduce Caffeine Intake

Drink Adequate Water

Enjoy Occasionally in Small Quantities

Fats, Oils, Sweets, Milk-based Foods, Cheese, Yogurt, Milk

Reduce Sodium Intake

Do Not Skip Meals

Drink Alcohol Only in Moderation

Enjoy Daily

Fish, Poultry, Meat, Eggs

Exercise Regularly

Read Food Labels

Legumes, Dried Peas, and Tofu

Starchy Vegetables

Always Handle, Cook, and Store Food Properly

Enjoy Daily at Most Meals

Whole-Grain Breads, Fortified Cereals, Rice, Brown Rice, Enriched Pasta

Dark Green Leafy Vegetables and Other Deeply Colored Vegetables

Calcium-Fortified 100% Juices; Dried, Fresh, or Frozen Fruits

Developed by Goulda A. Downer, Ph.D., R.D., C.N.S.
Metroplex Health and Nutrition Services, Inc., Washington, D.C. (2000)

that the emphasis on carbohydrates is similar, as is the direction to eat fewer sweets and fats. Along with the other dietary and lifestyle guidelines that are a part of the pyramid, Dr. Downer also stresses that you not skip meals; reduce your caffeine and sodium intake; drink plenty of water; and drink alcohol only in moderation. And you should still adhere to the serving sizes we'll tell you about later in the chapter.

The Vegetarian Food Pyramid

When you think of a vegetarian, you may think of a hippie in a Volkswagen minibus, but times have changed. More and more Black folks are becoming vegetarian, and they're as likely to be driving a Range Rover as a rust-bucket. In fact, many of our community's health advocates believe that African-Americans should be cutting back on meat and increasing the amount of plant-based foods in our diets. Some even recommend moving all the way to a vegetarian diet.

Research is starting to make a strong case for vegetarianism, moving it into the mainstream. Increasing numbers of studies show that vegetarians have a lower incidence of many chronic diseases than people who eat meat, and that a vegetarian diet can control some chronic health conditions. For instance, some studies show that a veggie diet can reduce hypertension in up to 75 percent of people with high blood pressure.

The reasons vegetarians seem to be so healthy are unclear. Is it because of the vegetarian diet itself? Are they generally more health-conscious? But no one can argue with the health benefits of loading your plate with fruits, vegetables, beans, legumes, and grains. A balanced vegetarian diet is typically lower in fat and calories, so it's a great way to lose and maintain your weight.

There are four common types of vegetarian:

• *Semivegetarian.* You probably thought that vegetarians only eat plant foods, but many semivegetarians eat most types of animal foods, including dairy products, eggs, fish, and poultry. The distinction is that they don't eat red meat (some semivegetarians won't eat poultry, either). Just note that most people who don't eat animal flesh at all don't consider semivegetarians "real" vegetarians. So if you're a semivegetarian, don't start bragging to your friends in front of someone who eats no animal flesh at all; they're likely to roll their eyes at you and take you to task for your meat-eating ways.

• *Lacto-ovo vegetarian.* These vegetarians will eat all dairy products and eggs, but won't eat animal flesh of any kind—not red meat, not poultry, not fish.

• *Lacto-vegetarian.* These vegetarians will eat dairy products, but no eggs or animal flesh of any kind.

• *Vegan.* Vegans eat no dairy products at all, nor will they eat animal flesh or any other product that comes from an animal (like eggs, butter, or honey). Some won't even *wear* any animal products (like leather shoes or wool).

Let's take a moment to look at the Vegetarian Food Pyramid. (Please do this whether you're vegetarian or not.) It's similar to the Ethnic Food Pyramid, except that animal flesh is excluded, and legumes, dried peas, beans, and soybeans are promoted to the base of the pyramid, to ensure that you get enough protein. These foods should be eaten at most meals, along with grains and vegetables.

To be enjoyed daily are fruits and juices; nonfat and low-fat yogurt and cheese, egg whites, and soy-based foods; and unsalted nuts and seeds and starchy vegetables.

Like the other pyramids, the top tier is to be enjoyed in small quantities and only occasionally. These foods include fats, oils, sweets, full-fat milks, cheeses, yogurts, and other milk-based foods.

The dietary and lifestyle recommendations are also a part of this pyramid.

Many people have the misconception that vegetarians can't get enough protein. While all types of vegetarians need to combine their foods to make sure they eat the full spectrum of amino acids, if they eat a balanced diet, they shouldn't have difficulty getting their protein. The exception is vegans, who have to be more conscious about what they eat since they eat no products from any animal at all. To be safe and to form complete proteins, Dr. Downer recommends that all vegetarians combine their plant-based foods during their meals, rather than risking that they'll forget to do so over the course of the day. That means they should eat their rice and beans together, not rice now and beans later. Other examples of food combining are given in the sidebar on page 66.

Vegetarian Food Pyramid

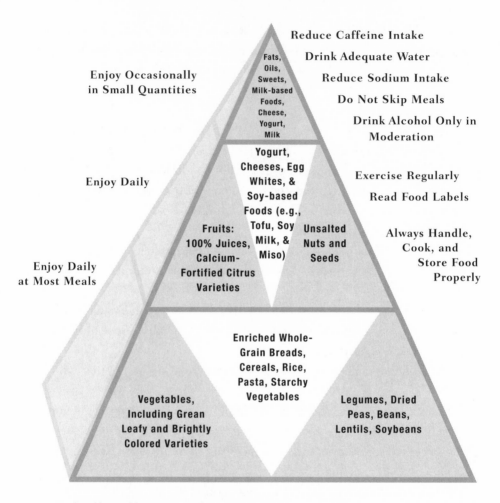

Reduce Caffeine Intake

Drink Adequate Water

Enjoy Occasionally in Small Quantities

Reduce Sodium Intake

Do Not Skip Meals

Drink Alcohol Only in Moderation

Fats, Oils, Sweets, Milk-based Foods, Cheese, Yogurt, Milk

Yogurt, Cheeses, Egg Whites, & Soy-based Foods (e.g., Tofu, Soy Milk, & Miso)

Enjoy Daily

Exercise Regularly

Read Food Labels

Fruits: 100% Juices, Calcium-Fortified Citrus Varieties

Unsalted Nuts and Seeds

Always Handle, Cook, and Store Food Properly

Enjoy Daily at Most Meals

Enriched Whole-Grain Breads, Cereals, Rice, Pasta, Starchy Vegetables

Vegetables, Including Green Leafy and Brightly Colored Varieties

Legumes, Dried Peas, Beans, Lentils, Soybeans

Developed by Goulda A. Downer, Ph.D., R.D., C.N.S.
Metroplex Health and Nutrition Services, Inc., Washington, D.C. (2000)

 The Right Stuff

It can't possibly be an accident that almost every indigenous civilization on the planet eats some version of rice and beans or peas—or that we intuitively combine peanut butter with bread; bean soup with rice, barley, or another grain; and

pasta with cheese. The science of combining plant-based foods to create a complete source of protein is ancient and intuitive.

You can turn an incomplete protein into a complete one by combining proteins with complementary foods that contain the missing amino acids. Try eating these combinations of food at every meal or during the course of the day:

Food	Combines With	Example
Grains	Legumes	Rice and peas or beans
	(or dairy products)	Macaroni and cheese
		Bread and peanut butter
Legumes	Nuts and seeds	Green beans and almonds
Nuts and seeds	Dairy products	Nuts and cheese
		Yogurt with trail mix

It's also important that vegetarians pay attention to the fat content of the protein sources they eat. Soy products, the only plant-based products to contain the full spectrum of amino acids and, therefore, very popular among vegetarians, can also be very high in fat. So look for low-fat soy milk and soy products. Nuts, another great protein source, are also high in fat. So while you should include them in your diet, don't eat them indiscriminately. Try to make beans and legumes your primary protein sources, instead.

And just because you're a vegetarian doesn't mean that you will automatically lose weight. Vegetarians can eat diets that are out of balance, just like everyone else. One example is junk-food vegetarians. They don't eat meat, but they don't eat a balanced diet, either. Surprised? A lot of young people eat this way, and a junk-food vegetarian can be just as unhealthy as anyone else.

Even if you're a healthy vegetarian, you need to eat foods in the proper proportions so your body gets the nutrients it needs. That means eating the proper portion sizes, which we'll tell you about shortly.

It may sound unthinkable to some, but more and more African-Americans are reconsidering how much meat they eat—and some are giving it up altogether. Those cheeseburgers and fried chicken legs may taste divine, but once all that saturated fat and cholesterol hits your bloodstream, in the words of B.B. King, the thrill is gone. Just cutting back on meat can trim a great deal of fat and cholesterol from your diet. And diets with high vegetable content are great for losing weight.

Myth 1: Getting enough protein is a problem for vegetarians.
Fact: Vegetarian diets—even those without dairy or eggs—can easily meet and exceed the RDA (recommended daily allowance) for protein. As long as vegetarians eat enough food to maintain weight and energy needs, they will have no problems with protein. In fact, it is nearly impossible to design a diet containing a variety of whole foods that is deficient in protein.

Myth 2: Vegetarians don't get enough iron.
Fact: Beans and leafy vegetables are excellent sources of iron. As with protein, meat-based diets supply more iron than most people need. The excess iron encourages the formation of free radicals, which can damage healthy cells, even turning them cancerous. A reasonable mix of vegetables and legumes—beans, lentils, and peas—supplies all the iron you need.

Myth 3: Dairy products are necessary for calcium.
Fact: Most greens—broccoli especially—are abundant sources of calcium. Not only do most vegetarians get enough calcium, they also absorb more calcium than meat-eaters because the excess protein obtained from a meat-based diet has been found to inhibit calcium absorption.

Myth 4: People were meant to eat meat.
Fact: The opposite is true. The small mouth, tooth structure (look at the difference between your dog's sharp fangs and your blunt teeth), large stomach, long small intestine, and puckered colon of human beings all suggest a physical structure designed for a plant-based, rather than a meat-based, diet. The human body's structure is much more like the vegetarian apes than that of meat-eating lions.

Myth 5: Vegetarians have low energy.
Fact: Fruits and vegetables are the best sources for complex carbohydrates, which provide lasting energy. Meat is totally lacking in such carbohydrates and contributes to sluggishness.

The Diabetes Soul Food Pyramid

If you suffer from diabetes, this is the pyramid for you. Developed by Constance Brown-Riggs, who is not only a registered dietitian but also a certified diabetes educator, the Diabetes Soul Food Pyramid offers a reasonable and effective approach to managing blood sugar.

If you are diabetic and considering using the Diabetes Soul Food Pyramid (or any other pyramid in *Lighten Up*) to lose weight, consult with your doctor beforehand and show him or her this program. Your doctor will be able to advise you on your best choices and your specific health-care needs. A registered dietitian (RD) or diabetes educator (CDE) can also help assist you so that you get the most out of the *HealthQuest* 30-Day Weight-Loss Program.

Although diabetics can eat the same foods as everyone else, the proportion of the diet that consists of carbohydrates is different. Carbohydrates affect the blood sugar more than any other nutrient, and carbohydrates are found in breads, cereals, fruits, vegetables, and dairy products. Eating too much of these foods at a meal or a snack can make the blood sugar elevate. To keep the blood sugar in check, diabetics should eat regular, more frequent—but smaller—meals and snacks. The

Diabetes Soul Food Pyramid

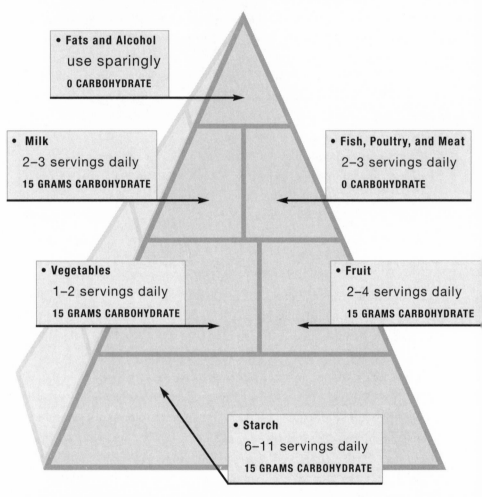

- **Fats and Alcohol**
  use sparingly
  0 CARBOHYDRATE

- **Milk**
  2–3 servings daily
  15 GRAMS CARBOHYDRATE

- **Fish, Poultry, and Meat**
  2–3 servings daily
  0 CARBOHYDRATE

- **Vegetables**
  1–2 servings daily
  15 GRAMS CARBOHYDRATE

- **Fruit**
  2–4 servings daily
  15 GRAMS CARBOHYDRATE

- **Starch**
  6–11 servings daily
  15 GRAMS CARBOHYDRATE

Source: © 1999 CBR Nutrition Enterprises

pyramid accounts for that as well as the fact that soul food is part of our diet—so you need not give up your cornbread and collard greens.

In addition to number of servings, the Diabetes Soul Food Pyramid incorporates carbohydrate guidelines: A carbohydrate choice is a serving of food from the starch, fruit, vegetable, or milk group; each serving gives you 15 grams of carbohydrate. Choose 3 to 4 carbohydrate choices at each meal, and 1 to 2 carbohydrate choices at planned snacks.

Here are the food categories, their carbohydrate amounts, and examples of servings of some typical soul foods that make up the pyramid tiers:

- **Fats and alcohol—SPARINGLY**
  0 CARBOHYDRATE
     1 teaspoon margarine or oil
     10 peanuts
     1 teaspoon lard
     1 slice bacon
     $\frac{1}{2}$ inch fatback
     2 tablespoons chitterlings

- **Milk—2 to 3 servings**
  15 GRAMS CARBOHYDRATE
     1 cup cow's milk
     1 cup goat's milk
     1 cup buttermilk
     $\frac{1}{2}$ cup evaporated milk

- **Fish, poultry, and meat—2 to 3 servings**
  0 CARBOHYDRATE
     2 to 3 ounces catfish, hog jowls, pig ear, neck bones, chicken, or goat

- **Vegetables—1 to 2 servings**
  15 GRAMS CARBOHYDRATE
     1 $\frac{1}{2}$ cups cooked kale, poke salad, collard greens, or turnips

- **Fruit—2 to 4 servings**
  15 GRAMS CARBOHYDRATE
     1 medium peach, apple, or orange
     1 $\frac{1}{4}$ cups watermelon
     17 muscadines
     $\frac{1}{2}$ cup orange or grapefruit juice

- **Starch—6 to 11 servings**
  15 GRAMS CARBOHYDRATE
    $1/2$ cup grits or cooked cereal
    1 biscuit (2 inches across)
    Cornbread (2-inch square)
    $1/2$ cup lima beans, black-eyed peas, or succotash
    $1/3$ cup yam, sweet potato, or rice

The Diabetes Soul Food Pyramid also includes healthful eating tips:

- Eat foods from each food group daily.
- If you are overweight, eat the lower number of servings from each group daily.
- Avoid too much fat.
- Eat fish, poultry, and lean meat more often than high-fat meat.
- Eat fresh fruits and vegetables daily.
- Avoid too much salt; do not add salt to your food after it is cooked.

Size Does Matter

When it comes to serving sizes, you can bet your bottom dollar, size does matter. You can eat the proper number of servings of the right types of foods, but if the serving sizes are too large, you'll consume too many calories and pick up weight.

We want to encourage you to monitor the amount of food you consume, but we'll also be honest and tell you that we live in a society that will make this effort very difficult. Capitalism is the reason why: Food manufacturers make more money when consumers eat more food, and companies are doing everything in their power to make that happen. Even though we need food to eat, the manufacturers' interests and our interests are somewhat at odds.

One very effective tool manufacturers use to get consumers to eat more food is to train us to look for "value" when we shop or go out to eat. When you think you're getting more food for less money, you feel good about yourself. But the more food that's available to us, the more many of us tend to eat. Ironically, while you're thinking you've made a good decision, you're also set up to gain more weight. Food manufacturers know this, of course, so they keep increasing the sizes of food that we buy. One of their greatest breakthroughs is the introduction of "supersize" items to fast-food menus. You see this same principle reflected in "family" or "bulk" sizes in the supermarket. Incidentally, food portions in sit-down restaurants are also getting larger.

Another example of manufacturers' effort to get us to eat more food is the sudden ubiquity of food. There used to be a time when food was available only at home, at the market, or in a restaurant. Now it's available everywhere, all the time. Take fast-food restaurants. Not only are they coming to a corner near you, they're also staying open later and later. Or note the introduction of fast-food franchises to malls, gas station minimarkets, and school cafeterias. Their presence is the result of a careful strategy.

As a result of this proliferation of food, Americans have lost their sense of how much to eat, how often to eat, and what constitutes a healthy portion size. And, unfortunately, as American food preferences are spreading around the world, so are the waistlines of Westernizing nations.

But if the food portions we've become accustomed to eating aren't good for us, what constitutes a healthy portion size?

"Servings of most foods will fit into the palm of an average woman's hand," says nutritionist Constance Brown-Riggs. Here's a list of single servings for each food group described in the USDA Food Guide Pyramid.

(Note: Some serving sizes of the Soul Food Pyramid and the Diabetes Soul Food Pyramid were given in their respective treatments earlier. Serving sizes for the Soul Food Pyramid, the Ethnic Food Pyramid, the Vegetarian Pyramid, and the Diabetes Soul Food Pyramid—even though their pyramid tier categories differ somewhat from one another and from the USDA pyramid—can be determined by using the recommended serving size for a particular food from the USDA Food Guide Pyramid guidelines that follow.)

Bread, Cereal, Rice, and Pasta Group

1 slice of bread

1 cup of ready-to-eat cereal

½ cup cooked cereal, rice, or pasta (½ cup rice or cereal fits into the palm of a woman's hand)

Vegetable Group

1 cup of raw, leafy vegetables (about the size of your fist)

½ cup of other veggies, cooked or raw

¾ cup of vegetable juice

Fruit Group

1 medium apple, orange, pear (the size of a baseball)

1 small banana

½ cup chopped, cooked, or canned fruit

¾ cup of fruit juice

Milk, Yogurt, and Cheese Group

1 cup milk or yogurt (lactose-free, enriched soy-milk, and fat-free or low-fat dairy products are all good choices)

1 ½ ounces of natural cheese, such as Cheddar (use fat-free or reduced-fat products most often)

2 ounces of processed cheese, such as American (again, go for the fat-free or reduced-fat options)

(One ounce of cheese is the equivalent of the size of your thumb from its tip to the first joint.)

Meat, Poultry, Fish, Dried Beans, Eggs, and Nuts Group

2 to 3 ounces of cooked lean meat, fish, or poultry

(Three ounces of meat is the equivalent of the size of a deck of cards, 10 one-inch cubes of meat, three meatballs the size of a golf ball, or one medium chicken leg.)

(One ounce of meat is the equivalent of ½ cup of tofu; 1 egg; ½ cup of cooked, dry beans; 2 ½ ounces of soy burger; 2 tablespoons of peanut butter; or ⅓ cup of nuts.)

FATS, OILS, AND SWEETS

1 teaspoon oil, mayonnaise, salad dressing, butter, or margarine

(One teaspoon is equivalent to the size of your thumb from its tip to the
first joint.)

Now that you know more about serving sizes, it's easy to see how it's
possible to eat the number of servings described on the food pyramids
without feeling stuffed—and that the range of servings provides enough
food to keep you full. A day of 6 to 11 servings of grains may seem like a
lot until you realize that a sandwich (2 slices of bread) is 2 servings in one
fell swoop. And depending upon your size and energy needs, you may
choose to stop at 6 servings or eat up to 11. Learning to control the sizes
of the portions you eat is an important aspect of a successful weight-loss
effort and is also crucial to maintaining your desired weight once you
reach it.

Deciding Which Pyramid to Use

Now that you've visited all the pyramids, it's time to decide which one
feels right to you. Don't sweat it: There's no right or wrong answer.
No matter which one you pick, you can't go wrong. (We told you we'd give
you choices, didn't we?) Here's how to choose:

Take another look at the various food pyramids presented in this chapter. Now look at your Food and Fitness Diary, and compare the foods that
you ate when you did the week-long food-tracking exercise to the food
groups of the various pyramids. Note how many servings of grains, meats,
vegetables, fruits, snacks, and other foods that you ate, and any other
food patterns. Now consider the following:

Which of the five food pyramids—the USDA Food Guide Pyramid,
the Soul Food Pyramid, the Ethnic Food Pyramid, the Vegetarian
Pyramid, or the Diabetes Soul Food Pyramid—contains more of the
foods that you typically eat? You should be able to draw some conclusions
that will help you choose which pyramid may be right for you. Then just
follow your hunch (based, of course, on your food likes and patterns) and
pick the one that feels right. Don't fret; know that you can change your
mind later on.

All Pyramids Are Not Alike

You'll notice that some foods fit on one layer of one pyramid but are on a different layer of another pyramid. For example, the USDA Food Guide Pyramid has milk, yogurt, and cheese together on the third tier (from the base) of the pyramid, while the Ethnic Food Pyramid has milk, yogurt, and cheese on the top tier. Likewise, some daily servings are different: the USDA Food Guide Pyramid recommends 3 to 5 servings of vegetables, while the Diabetes Soul Food Pyramid recommends 1 to 2 servings.

The pyramids really are not interchangeable. You should not mix and match the pyramids throughout your week; that is, don't use the USDA Food Guide Pyramid on Monday, then switch to the Soul Food Pyramid on Tuesday, then the Ethnic Food Pyramid for the remainder of the week. And certainly do not switch pyramids within the same day, using one set of guidelines for breakfast, lunch, and snacks, then finishing off your day with a different set of guidelines for dinner. Stick with the same pyramid for the entire thirty-day program. If you feel you'd like to switch pyramids, and try a different pyramid after thirty days, by all means, do so.

Now, if none of these pyramids feels comfortable—because your diet doesn't even come close to their recommendations—there's no need to get upset; you're not alone. Like many Americans, you probably don't eat enough fruits and vegetables, and eat too many carbohydrates, meats, dairy products, and sweets. Still, choose a pyramid that represents how you'd ideally like to eat, now that you understand the role that a proper diet plays in weight loss.

If you suffer from heart disease, cancer, or any chronic disease other than diabetes, any of these food pyramids should work for you because they limit the amount of fat, calories, and sodium in your diet. But talk to your doctor to see if there's anything special about your condition that requires you to make other changes. For instance, some studies suggest that a vegetarian diet may be better if you suffer from many chronic diseases, including heart disease and cancer—or at least a diet containing more fruits and vegetables than are depicted in any but the Vegetarian Pyramid.

Make That Change!

Congratuations! You're well on your to a healthier, more fit you. Believe it or not, you know enough to begin to adjust your diet. Move slowly by taking baby steps. For instance, if you don't eat enough fruit, start to eat an apple for breakfast and an orange when your energy drops during midafternoon. Skip the french fries at lunch and order a small salad, instead (but go light on the dressings—you know they are often loaded with fat). If you regularly cook with shortening, bacon grease, palm oil, or lard, start to reduce the amount of fat in your diet by substituting broth, bouillon, and seasonings. In chapter 6 we'll provide you with some healthier alternatives to frying your food, but for now, you may want to cut back on the amount of oil you use and start using olive oil or another unsaturated oil more often. By gradually changing your diet to reflect the guidelines provided by the food pyramids, you will naturally increase the number of fruits, veggies, and grains you eat, while decreasing fats, oils, sweets, and animal products. So don't be surprised if you start to lose weight without much additional effort.

Now that you're starting to make changes to your diet, we want to make sure to tell you that we don't want you to feel like you're on some strict dietary regimen—you're not. While we want you to begin to look to a food pyramid for guidance, we don't want you thinking that any food is a "bad" food. *No type of food is prohibited from your diet.* To prove this, take a look at the food list in appendix 1. This list illustrates the wide variety of foods that are available to you. You'll find just about everything there, from chicken chow mein to broccoli, from pork chops and cabbage to pecan pie and cantaloupe. All foods are there because—unless you have a health-related dietary restriction—all foods are available to you. The key, as we stated earlier, is Size Matters. *Do not* deprive yourself, but eat in the right portions and with a sense of nutrition. We hope you feel empowered by everything you learned and will be better able to make conscious dietary decisions because you understand the impact your choices have on your weight and health.

We encourage you to enjoy every food you eat, no matter the occasion—whether you're enjoying breakfast with the Sunday paper or late-night dessert and coffee after going to a show. Always *enjoy* your food. We want you to savor the way hot tomato soup warms your insides, delight yourself with key lime pie from time to time, let watermelon juice trickle down your chin. Just make an effort to consume the foods at the top of the pyramid sparingly.

Nonetheless, if you're like the rest of us, what you ate this morning for breakfast is probably substantially different from what your great-great-grandparents ate 150 years ago—not to mention what your African ancestors ate for centuries before that. Many experts suggest that to lose weight and become healthier, we need to return to something closer to the ancestral diet described in the introduction. We need to change our habits and go back to basics. By doing so, we also recapture an important part of our heritage.

"African-Americans need to return to a more natural way of eating," Dr. Carolyn Coker-Ross stated in an interview in *HealthQuest* magazine. "Eating fresh, like our ancestors did, gives a continuity of culture for our children, so they'll grow up knowing what collard greens and snap peas are." Knowledge can be powerful food for thought.

And we need to focus on being healthy—not solely on being thin. "Americans think being fit is being thin, but being thin does not always mean that you are fit or healthy," she adds. (See the section on eating disorders on page 86.)

We have a huge advantage over many of our ancestors. We have the power to make choices about the foods we eat. Most of us are fortunate enough that we no longer eat merely to survive. We eat for pleasure, for health, for satisfaction, for spiritual renewal. And because we have choices, we also have the power—and the responsibility—to build a diet that contributes to our physical, emotional, and spiritual well-being.

Think It Through

What shape do you think your pyramid is? Most Americans, if we were to draw the pyramid categories to represent our eating habits, would likely draw a shape resembling a square, an hourglass, or one that may even be a little top-heavy, perhaps even be a pyramid but be fully upside down.

Go back to your food diary and draw your own personal pyramid—not the way you wish it looked, but the way it actually looks. Keep all the food categories where they are, but increase or decrease their size based on how you eat. For instance, if you eat a lot of greasy snacks or sweets, draw a larger crown, so your personal pyramid may be top-heavy. If you love hamburgers and slather cheese all over your food, your pyramid may resemble an hourglass.

Start to think of ways to get your pyramid to be structurally sound. Write your ideas in your food diary. Perhaps you can begin to think of ways to adapt some of your favorite recipes, or to add more balance to your diet by incorporating some healthy snacks. Let the food-tracking self-assessment exercise, and your personal pyramid that you're about to draw, help inform you of your food preferences and habits. Then get to work on making that pyramid the solid, lasting temple it was meant to be.

For Your Spirit

Next time you eat a healthy meal and have some quiet time to yourself, allow yourself to get in touch with the power of every food you eat. As you chew, sense that your food is performing an important job in your body. Each time you bite into a low-fat carbohydrate, pat yourself on the back for choosing to bring a healthy source of energy into your body. Know that it is regulating your blood sugar, helping with digestion and protecting you against cancer, diabetes and heart disease. When you chew a bite of protein, feel good about the fact that you're making and rejuvenating new cells and muscles. As each bite of food travels across your tongue, down your esophagus, and into your stomach, allow yourself to feel the power that comes from making healthy choices. Do this whenever you feel good about the foods you're eating.

CHAPTER 5

Getting into the Right Head

Exploring Eating and Feelings, Size and Self-Image

Tradition and habit explain a great deal of what we eat every day. Many of our dietary habits are just that—habits—that have solidified over years of repetition. They become so ingrained that we hardly know why we do them anymore.

Say your mother fed you pork chop sandwiches when you were a sprout and you loved them. Now you fix them for yourself and you love them still. Is it simply the taste that sends you to the meat counter and then to the frying pan?

Often the mental and emotional associations we make with a food have a lot to do with why that food is so appealing. Food can symbolize an awful lot. Maybe your mom knew pork chop sandwiches were your daddy's favorite lunch, and she would slip one in his lunchbox every now and then when he wasn't expecting it. When he got home, you'd watch him give her a big kiss and tell her how good those chops were. And they'd both be in a good mood for the rest of the evening. It was a pleasant memory—a memory that's still there, somewhere in the back of your mind, when you're savoring a pork chop sandwich today.

You can see how a simple sandwich can bring into the picture all sorts of complex images and feelings—family, love, comfort, community, togetherness, protection, happiness. It's these mental and emotional associations we make with food that explain why many of us turn to familiar "comfort" foods in times of crisis—when we get a terrible performance rating at work, for example, or when a cherished relationship breaks down. Which is also why it can be challenging to even *think* about altering what we eat. ("Sure, I can change my diet. No problem. But if I don't fix my famous macaroni and cheese for Sunday dinner, well, my family will wonder what's wrong.") And even when we're committed to our diets, an emotional setback or just a stressful day can nudge us off the wagon. ("Those folks at work got on my last nerve today; I *deserve* a bowl of ice cream.")

But when we use food as an emotional pacifier to help us cope with despair, loneliness, or other pain, it can lead to uncontrolled weight—especially if the pain is ongoing and we aren't coping with it in any other way besides eating, and the food isn't all that nutritious. Deborah, a Seattle artist (not her real name), spoke openly in *HealthQuest* magazine about her long struggle to come to peace with food.

"My problem with food and body image began in childhood. I was a chubby child, a slim teenager, then an overweight adult," she says. As a young teen, her parents' warnings about her weight convinced her to diet. "I thought my life would be better if I were thin," she recalls. "In that sense, thinness meant love and acceptance." Still, she had to sort through confusing mixed messages about food. "Eat this wonderful decadent food, but don't get overweight," her parents seemed to say.

By the time Deborah had reached her late twenties, she had lost and regained the same fifty pounds—and then some. She'd tried several weight-loss programs, some successfully, others less so. "It never occurred to me that I was pretty much avoiding my feelings. I had lost touch with myself. Food was companionship and entertainment. It became a senses-dulling drug.

"Some time ago I learned to mask my emotions—my pain, anger, and frustration—with food," she says. "Instead of expressing my true feelings, or asking for what I wanted and needed, I had another cookie. Food helped me blot out my feelings."

Food and Feelings

Deborah's story is not unusual. We know, of course, that it's best to eat when we're hungry. But often our emotional state—anxiousness, worry, or even happiness—can tempt us to eat more than we need or when we're not really hungry. For example, researchers have found that men especially tend to overeat when they're celebrating. Women, on the other hand, often have favorite snacks they turn to when they're feeling "hormonal" or down.

There are those people who tend to eat when they're bored. If they can't turn to some fun or constructive activity, they open the cabinets or the refrigerator (or both) and eat as if it were a hobby. These folks are related to the "sensory eaters," people who crave foods that tantalize their senses. They get pleasure from the smooth and creamy texture of a bowl of pudding or the crisp crackle of potato chips. Of course, we all have our favorite foods and enjoy crunching popcorn or licking an ice-cream cone. But if food seems to have become your primary source of pleasure, it may mean that you lack other pleasures or activities in your life. In that case, cutting down on your commitments and taking up a hobby may help you keep from picking up extra weight.

You've probably known someone who can't seem to touch a thing to eat when they're nervous or worried. But there are as many folks—perhaps you're one of them—who do just the opposite. Not only do they eat when they're nervous, lonely, or depressed, they eat more than ever. Often, their eating is almost unconscious—they're so distracted by their concern about their mother's illness or their argument with their spouse that they're barely aware of what they're putting in their mouth.

In fact, this may be the case with most instances of "emotional" eating: We're so wrapped up in our mental state—be it happiness or despair—that we're not paying attention to what we're eating. Paradoxically, the key may be to focus more on what's going on in your life—notice when you tend to binge. Is it when you're nervous? When you're angry, or frustrated? Or do you throw caution to the wind when things are going particularly well and you feel as though you deserve a treat? If you can trace the pattern of your overeating, you will have taken one step toward being able to eat with more awareness during those "times of temptation."

Review the "Think It Through" exercise that you did in chapter 3, and see if you can pinpoint any patterns that lead you to overeat and to make poor food choices; conversely, are there things that you did that helped you maintain, or regain, your "control"? Strive for "mindful" eating, where you are aware of your hunger and are enjoying your foods and the beneficial aspects of your healthier life, with it's structured yet flexible eating plan. Avoid the "mindless" eating, where you are eating and choosing your foods based on the destructive thoughts and circumstances that prevent you from attaining your goals. You, like our ancestors who endured much harsher life circumstances, are endowed with a bottomless reservoir of strength. Tap into it and use it.

Big and Beautiful?: Examining Size and Self-Image

Food and feelings are intrinsically linked to how we feel about ourselves and our self-image. Until recent years, African-Americans have had a different idea about what it means to have a beautiful body.

In some cultures in Africa, being physically weighty symbolized prosperity and health. It meant you had the means to eat well and live a leisurely lifestyle—you didn't burn off those calories by working too hard.

Meanwhile, in this country, as Southern belles were squeezing themselves into wasp-waisted corsets, our sisters in the kitchen had more important things to worry about. In the bad old days of slavery and segregation, being small might be read as being weak and make you the target for unwanted attention. For Black women, being heavy symbolized a tough, powerful exterior, a means to resist assault. It also meant a little extra padding against the cold, a cushioned hug for those you loved, a body that could make it in the fields from before dawn until after dark.

Then, too, whoever made up the old saying, "Men like meat, dogs like bones," was probably a brother—and he wasn't talking about chuck steak. A Black man wanted a woman with something to hold on to. And vice versa. On men, extra pounds meant power, strength, and some measure of protection. That extra bulk was likely to ensure he, too, could work hard, and thus be a good provider for the family.

We're talking in past tense here, but in some cases those considerations remain today. In fact, one study showed that ovulating women found strong-looking men more attractive than their smaller, gentler-looking counterparts. (Scientists think it has something to do with subconsciously picking the person who looked as if he had the stronger genes.)

So, if being big has had so many advantages for Black folks, why are we now so obsessed with losing weight?

Images of beauty change from decade to decade. At the turn of the century and again in the forties and fifties, the ideal female figure was a lush one. In the twenties and the sixties, narrow, boyish shapes were in. When Black people started being part of mainstream America, we began to be affected by these changing images as well. With the advent of movies and television and access to the proliferation of fashion magazines (and more leisure time to read them), we began to be bombarded by images of beauty that didn't reflect our dark skin, kinky hair, and broad features. When we did see Black folks who were considered beautiful, they often were sepia-toned versions of White models and movie stars: light-skinned, fine-boned, svelte, and perfectly proportioned. (Think Dorothy Dandridge, Lena Horne, Harry Belafonte.)

Later, there was the advent of the fitness craze. Remember when aerobics hit the scene? The goal was good health but, judging by the typical aerobics instructor, you had to have a blond ponytail and be able to fit into a leotard to get there. It was a brave sister who would squeeze her few extra pounds into spandex and go jump around in a room with a big mirror. And in front of *other people*, no less.

Today, even though we're seeing our Black selves reflected more in the media, it's a triumph with a hidden message that plagues us. We celebrate our Black Miss Americas, supermodels, athletes, and movie stars, but they, too, seem to reinforce that thin-is-in image. Think about it: You've never seen Denzel Washington or Vanessa Williams with an ounce of fat, have you?

We live in a nation where the icon for beauty is thinness, and tall thinness at that—a gold standard that, for most of us, is about as possible to achieve as reaching inside of our bodies and rearranging our genes. In a culture that's positively consumed with physical appearance, it's all too easy to get swept up in the media frenzy that dictates what's beautiful and what's not. From *Vogue* to *Ally McBeal* to the Victoria's Secret catalog, the message is loud and clear: The world's most beautiful women are tall, thin, billowy blondes with subtle curves in all the right places. (For men, the image is similar. Just replace the curves with a rippling stomach and bulging biceps.) If you can't be tall and blond, then at least be thin.

In fact, only about 5 percent of the population can claim a body size like supermodel Tyra Banks or actress Halle Barry. (Need proof? Just watch the people sitting on the bus with you or walking down the sidewalk beside you. How often do you see a perfectly gorgeous five-foot-ten, 120-pound woman?) But we get bombarded with so many pictures of waiflike models that all that psychological conditioning convinces us that a size 6 is the norm. It's not, of course. Can you guess what size the average American woman wears? Size 8? Think bigger. Size 10? Come again. It's *size 14*. But if we think size 6 is the norm, our size is then, by definition, *abnormal*. The competing images of what we *should* look like versus what we *do* look like can weigh heavily on us.

Our Place in the World

Many of us yearn to be smaller, if only to fit more comfortably into a world that was designed for thinner people. For some of us, these concerns began in childhood, when Mama headed straight for the "husky" rack to pick out our school clothes. For others, it started once puberty kicked in, when our so-called baby fat (a fourteen-year-old baby?) settled into plus-sized hips and thighs. For many mothers among us, it happened during pregnancy; that little bundle of giggles left us carrying twenty extra hard-to-get-rid-of pounds.

"You've got to understand. I've never been a normal size," Dena (not her real name) explained to *HealthQuest*. "I went straight from size 6X to size 16, then to 24 and 26, and right on up."

The twenty-three-year-old has been struggling to lose weight as long as she can remember. She can't remember the last time she stepped on a scale, but she's pretty sure she weighs more than 350 pounds.

"Even as a child I was overweight," she says. "Doctors and my family alike told me I'd eventually lose my 'baby fat.' Well, I didn't."

Dena often thinks no one understands her weight dilemma. But many of us do. We've been there. It's true that Black folks make allowances when it comes to body weight. We compliment Sister Emma on the new, size 24 dress she bought for the church banquet. We don't blink when Roy complains that his Electra 225 is getting too small for him to fit behind the wheel. Yet people also make negative assumptions about us because of our size. You've heard it:

"Now, she knows she doesn't need to be making a second trip to the buffet table."

"Why would he get a Big Mac and a milkshake?"

"She's got such a pretty face . . . if she'd just lose some of that weight."

We begin to internalize all that we hear. For those of us who are carrying extra weight, it's as if we can hear people whispering about us. *If only he didn't eat so much*, people must be thinking when they see us. *She could be so happy if she was smaller*, they seem to say in their covert stares. To those of us on the receiving end of that negative attention, it doesn't really much matter that Africans value bigness as a sign of prosperity, or that African-Americans see it as a sign of power. We've heard the insults, we know the sting of rejection, we've seen the sad stares. We know full well that being big can hurt.

It doesn't take long for this stigma of obesity to chip away at our self-esteem. Soon we can see ourselves only through a "fat" lens—one that distorts everything about us. We're so focused on our physical size that we can't appreciate how wonderful we are in other ways. You may be smart, but your intellect can't seem to make up for your size. You may be quite fashionable, but you won't be able to accept a genuine compliment. You might be generous, talented, funny, fair—God's gift to the planet—but all that will be muffled under the emotional weight of being bigger than you want to be.

Yes, maybe Mavis, the waitress at our favorite greasy spoon, knows our order by heart (*"Hey, Marvin! Double meatloaf platter, extra gravy!"*). Maybe we *have* parked in front of the movie of the week and polished off almost half a chocolate cake—or a whole bag of nacho chips or all but one in the box of glazed donuts. But figuring out *why* we eat the way we do is the ultimate riddle.

When Losing Becomes an Obsession

Given the role that body type plays in our image-oriented culture, it's easy to understand how some people's concern about losing weight can turn into an obsession. We don't hear much about African-

Americans' weight-loss frustrations snowballing into eating disorders, but it's clear that eating disorders among Black women are relatively common.

When *Essence* magazine asked its readers to analyze how they felt about their eating habits, 52 percent of respondents said they were preoccupied with food, 38 percent said they go on eating binges they can't stop, and 30 percent revealed that the thought of food literally controls their lives. These results suggest that eating disorders may be much more prevalent in the Black community than we like to admit. And if sisters engage in eating binges—the practice of eating large amounts of food for at least two days a week for at least six months—at the rate indicated in the *Essence* survey, this behavior could be partly responsible for the high prevalence of obesity among Black women.

You've also probably heard of anorexia nervosa and bulimia, and may have assumed that these eating disorders are also a "White-girl thing." But Black folks suffer from these problems, too. (Most sufferers tend to be women.) An anorexic patient usually has an unrealistic fear of becoming fat—and thin is never thin enough—so she consequently eats very little. She obsesses over calories, skips meals, and sometimes uses laxatives or diuretics to increase her weight loss. A person with bulimia binges on enormous amounts of high-calorie foods only to "purge" the calories with laxatives or through self-induced vomiting. Both anorexia and bulimia can lead to very serious health problems and ultimately can be fatal.

If you engage in these behaviors or experience the symptoms, the HealthQuest 30-Day Weight-Loss Program is not for you. Engaging in our program, or in any diet not supervised by a health-care practitioner, could cause you serious physical harm. Consult your doctor or a therapist, instead. Both disorders can be treated with diet counseling and antidepressant medication. The most successful techniques involve psychotherapy.

Think It Through

Here's a self-image exercise. It works best if you disrobe at least partially. Find a full-length mirror and spend one or two minutes really looking at yourself. Start at the top of your head and follow each line and curve of your body down to the soles of your feet. Notice the slope of your shoulders, the contours of your stomach, how your skin fits around your legs and arms. Try to imagine never having seen yourself before, and notice aspects of your body as if for the very first time. Don't start judging what's good or bad about what you see. Just write down what you see in the mirror, especially anything you've never noticed before.

Now, starting at the top of your head and working your way down to your feet, write down what you like and what you would change about your body. Don't just include hips, thighs, and stomach, but hair, eyes, ankles, hands—every part of you.

Next, picture your body after you successfully lose weight. Visualize what will happen to the features you noticed in the mirror. Write down the things that will change.

> How many things on your original list will change when you complete this diet?
> How many things could change without you having to diet?
> How many things can't be changed? (Skin color, the shape of your hands.)
> How many are hereditary? (You've got your mother's bone structure. Your father's ankles.)

This exercise gives you a chance to really see yourself for who you are physically, and to learn to live with and appreciate the things about you that are a legacy of your family or something that you're actually proud of.

For Your Spirit

Our vision of ourselves is very powerful. It affects how proudly we stand, how clearly we speak, whether we look someone in the eye or not. The more you see yourself as powerful, confident, talented, worthy, the more you'll act out those traits. If you don't see it, you won't be it. That's the point of visualizing your ideal self: Envisioning change is the first step to making it happen. You have to first see it in your mind.

Every dieter who visualizes an "after" body, pictures a different image. For you that may mean a tighter tummy, firmer thighs, and so on. The diet and fitness regimen in your thirty-day program is designed to help you move in that direction.

But it's important, too, to have a realistic goal—and to separate what a diet can do from what it can't. It's not enough to think of this journey as a physical makeover—something any decent plastic surgeon might be able to handle. Sure you can have a tighter tummy, but losing weight won't make you taller. It won't narrow your nose or make your hair grow. Dieting can make you thinner, but unless that's your only criteria for beauty, it won't make you beautiful or self-confident.

Beauty, confidence, and self-acceptance go hand in hand. And they start in your mind. So along with losing a few here and tightening up a little there, during your diet you're going to work on coming to new levels of self-acceptance as well.

Part of the journey is *recognizing who you are*—the part of you that doesn't change no matter how much weight you gain or lose. And part of it is learning to feel better about that real you. That means coming to understand, really understand, without question that the person you really are was Divinely created and, therefore, just perfect.

Oddly enough, the first step toward changing yourself is to start truly accepting yourself as you are. There's something about self-acceptance that takes the pressure off and allows you to move toward your goals with greater ease. It's as if you're not so much changing, but effortlessly evolving toward being the person you're destined to be.

So, for starters, think again about those physical and nonphysical traits that you feel good about. Maybe it's your smile, your attractive hands, your unselfishness, your talent for playing the piano, your efficiency at work. Make a list in your diary. That's what it's for.

Now look for ways to focus more attention on the things you really like about yourself. If you play the piano well, spend more time at the keyboard. If your smile is beautiful, use it more often. You're a giver? A hard worker? Sign up for a volunteer opportunity or a new project at work.

Take every opportunity to give thanks for something wonderful about yourself. No, we're not trying to make you conceited or vain; being thankful for your gifts and talents isn't vanity. You may find saying a word of thanks makes you more humble, more grateful, and more willing to use your gifts for good.

Strengthening Affirmations

Using affirmations—positive words you say to yourself or aloud— can be a powerful tool to help you in your daily efforts. Remember, the more you use an affirmation, the sooner it will become a belief. Repeat these affirmations as often as you can.

Acceptance Affirmation

Look again at your list of the things you listed as hereditary or that won't be affected by weight loss (height, breast size, and so on). Say this affirmation:

These are the traits that I was born with. God* gave me these character- istics for a reason. I don't look like anyone else, and I'm proud of my indi- viduality.

*Of course, you can say "Allah," "Jehovah," "the Creator," "the Universe"—whatever term is comfortable for you. Or say "I have these characteristics for a reason."

Self-Love Affirmation

Look at your list again. Copy the list of things you like about your body onto a separate small piece of paper, and tape it to your closet door or mirror. When you bathe or get dressed and before you go to bed, read the list and say the following affirmation:

I really love these things about myself. These are some of my most attrac- tive physical traits, but I am attractive and beautiful in many ways, inside and out. I am thankful for the gifts I have been given.

CHAPTER 6

Making the Health Connections

Your Weight, Body Mass Index, Waist-Hip Ratio, and Family Medical History

Much in the same way our dietary habits are linked to our ancestral heritage, our weight, shape, and health are linked to our genetics and family history. Understanding your family medical history will help you to understand the kinds of obstacles you're up against when trying to lose weight, and will also inform you of food choices and activity changes that will be beneficial to your success in the program. But before we delve deeper into that area—and start getting even more serious about losing weight—let's see how much of your weight is *healthy*. This will give you some idea of how much weight you might want to lose.

Determining Your Body Mass Index (BMI) and Waist-Hip Ratio

As you've probably figured out by now, determining how much you should weigh is no longer as simple as looking at a height-weight chart. Although your weight in numbers is important, it's only one part of the story. The amount of fat that you carry is the critical measurement— one that can be more useful to African-Americans than any comparison to an "ideal" weight. It's also important to know where on your body you carry that weight.

Body Mass Index (BMI)

To determine how much of your body is made of fat, calculate your Body Mass Index (BMI). Unlike a bathroom scale, which only depicts your weight, the BMI reflects body weight in proportion to stature. It can give you a fairly accurate assessment of how much of your body is composed of fat. For women, a healthy BMI is between 20 and 28. Said another way, 20 to 28 percent of the body of a healthy women should be composed of fat. For men, it should be between 15 and 22. Obesity is defined as having a BMI of 30 or higher. The following formula is a simple way to calculate your BMI:

$$BMI = weight \text{ (in pounds)} \div height \text{ (in inches)}^2 \times 705.$$

Here's how a woman who is five-foot-six (66 inches tall) and weighs 150 pounds would calculate her BMI:

$$BMI = 150 \text{ pounds} \div (66)^2 \times 705$$
$$BMI = 150 \text{ pounds} \div 4356 \times 705$$
$$BMI = 24.27$$

Our fictional woman's BMI is 24.27. Said another way, approximately 24 percent of her body is composed of fat. This is well within the healthy range for a woman.

You can also use the following chart to determine if you are at a healthy weight. The weight ranges shown are for adults. While they are not exact ranges of healthy and unhealthy weights, they will give you a sense of your range, and if you are at health risk for complications associated with overweight and obesity.

Weigh yourself without clothes, then find your weight on the bottom of the graph. Go straight up from that point until you come to the line that matches your height (without shoes). Then look to find your weight group.

Healthy Weight = BMI between 18.5 and 25
Overweight = BMI between 25 and 30
Obese = BMI of 30 and higher

Waist-Hip Ratio

In addition to what percentage of your body weight is fat, where you carry your weight also has significance for your health. People who tend to put

Body Mass Index

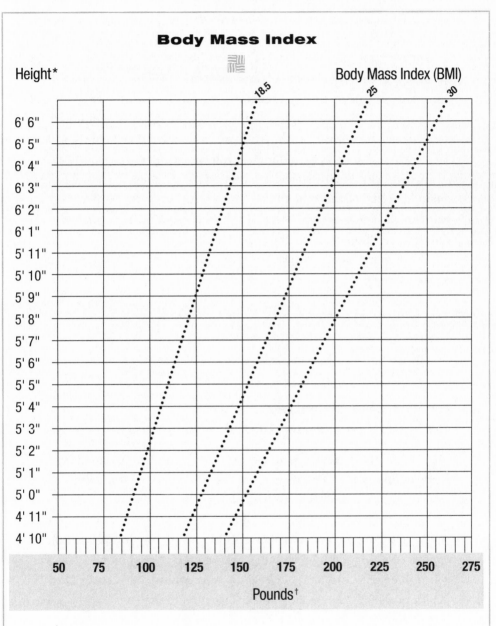

* Without shoes.
† Without clothes.

Source: Report of the Dietary Guidelines Advisory Committee on the Dietary
Guidelines for Americans, 2000.

on weight about the waist—"apple-shaped" people, may have a greater chance of developing high levels of "bad" cholesterol, hardening of the arteries (which causes the blood vessels in the heart to harden and become narrow, reducing blood flow), high blood pressure, and diabetes. "Pear-shaped" people carry their extra weight below the waistline and don't seem to have as high a risk of developing the conditions that "apples" do. A healthy waist-hip ratio for women is .80 or below; for men 1.0 or below. Here's how to calculate your waist-hip ratio for yourself:

Measure around the smallest part of your waistline—don't pull in, just stand relaxed. For this example, assume you are a woman with a 34-inch waist. Next, measure your hips at the largest point. Let's assume this number is 43 inches.

Then, divide the waist measurement by the hip measurement. For this example:

$$34 \div 43 = .79$$

The woman in this example fits into the healthy range.

Doing the Numbers: Calculating Your Ideal Weight

Now is the time to get down to business and start crunching the numbers. The following exercises will help you determine where you currently are and where you need to be. You'll learn if you are within a healthy weight range and, if not, how much weight your BMI indicates you need to lose. If you are within a healthy weight range, does the shape of your body suggest that you need to take preventive measures (such as a healthier diet and an exercise program) against developing chronic health problems like cardiovascular disease and diabetes? Think about these after you've done your numbers.

In your Food and Fitness Diary, take a page and mark today's date and calculate a few easy figures. These will help you plan your goals and give you a baseline to compare your results against. Write in your answers to the following:

1. Determine your ideal weight according to the BMI chart in this chapter. Write in the following two entries:

   My present weight: _____
   My "ideal" weight: _____

2. Find your body mass index (BMI) using the chart in this chapter. Write in the following two entries:

   My present BMI: _____
   Healthy BMI <u>18.5–25</u>

3. Determine your body shape using the waist-hip ratio equation in this chapter. Write in the following four entries:

   Waist in inches: _____
   Hips in inches: _____
   Waist inches divided by hip inches: _____
   Body shape: Apple [ ]   Pear [ ]   In between [ ]

Think It Through

By assessing who in your family has what health conditions, you can better determine what diseases are hereditary and whether or not you're at risk for them.

In your Food and Fitness Diary, set up a chart of the illnesses listed below. Then list all of the people in your family, living and deceased, who have (or had) the illnesses given in the chart. Also list their current age, their current health, and whether or not obesity is a factor in their life, now or at some previous time. Try to trace back several generations on both sides of the family. Start with your immediate family (parents and siblings); then look at your grandparents, aunts, and uncles; followed by great-grandparents, great-aunts, and great-uncles. You'll probably need to enlist the help of several relatives.

When it's completed, take it with you on your next visit to your doctor or health-care practitioner and ask to have the results interpreted with you. Your doctor should be able to draw conclusions and offer suggestions for what you should (and shouldn't) be doing to maintain your health and well-being.

 Making the Connection to Family Health

By Jimmie Briggs

"I don't know," was Fannie Moore-Murray's typical response during medical exams when asked by the doctor what illnesses were present in her family. That changed ten years ago when she discovered genealogy, the study of family history. Preparing to retire after thirty-six years working for the city of Philadelphia, Murray started thinking about how to spend her postemployment life.

"I went to a family reunion conference here in the city and ended up joining the African-American Genealogy Group, by accident," she recalls. "I believed like many others do that African-Americans can't research their roots."

In the process of chronicling five generations of her family's history, from its Georgia roots to the present, she also found legacies of heart disease, high blood pressure, and hypertension being passed down from one generation to the next.

"Life hasn't been the same since," says Murray.

Advances in computer technology and genealogical resources are helping many Black people trace their roots and piece together family history they thought had been destroyed by slavery. In the process, many people stumble across medical predispositions that run through branches of their family. Some document this history in a medical family tree, then use the information to change their lifestyles before the same health problems that plagued their older relatives threaten their well-being, too.

"If you don't know your medical roots from going back and getting your family's history, you lose out," explains Laura Chapman, president of the central Florida chapter of the Afro-American Historical and Genealogical Society. As she was compiling a historical record of her mother's family, she discovered a pattern of heart attacks among the men. All of her uncles except one died of heart disease and her own brother died of a heart attack following an earthquake in San Francisco. Hypertension was rampant among men and women.

"I wanted my daughters to know the things that fall within my family and their father's family," says Chapman. "One daughter is overweight and has done an excellent job with her nutrition. I don't frighten them, but they need to be aware of what could happen and try to prevent them. Families should be [mindful] beforehand, not when a relative is half-dead. You have people come to say, 'Yeah, Uncle Willie had the same thing happen to him.' Well, why didn't you say something before the person started feeling this way?"

Even people who already have an ailment can begin the process of making lifestyle changes. Many get motivated when they discover that they're suffering from the same diseases that killed their ancestors.

"With high blood pressure and heart disease in my family, I make an extra effort to exercise," notes Moore-Murray. "Three times a week I go to the Y and am aware of certain things in my diet, because I do have a heart problem. My children and grandchildren are aware of my research."

Whenever Moore-Murray sees a doctor now, she always has something to say.

"I wanted to know more about my family than anyone else in the world," she says. "And now I can say that I do."

Family Health History Chart

HEART DISEASE (INCLUDING ANY HEART CONDITIONS)

Who?	Current age?	Condition/Current health?	Obese?
_____	_____	_____	_____
_____	_____	_____	_____
_____	_____	_____	_____

HYPERTENSION

Who?	Current age?	Current health?	Obese?
_____	_____	_____	_____
_____	_____	_____	_____
_____	_____	_____	_____

DIABETES

Who?	Current age?	Current health?	Obese?
_____	_____	_____	_____
_____	_____	_____	_____
_____	_____	_____	_____

CANCER—BREAST, COLON, LUNG, PROSTATE, OVARIAN, OTHER

Who?	Current age?	Type/Current health?	Obese?
_____	_____	_____	_____
_____	_____	_____	_____
_____	_____	_____	_____

KIDNEY PROBLEMS

Who?	Current age?	Current health?	Obese?
_____	_____	_____	_____
_____	_____	_____	_____
_____	_____	_____	_____

ARTHRITIS

Who?	Current age?	Type/Current health?	Obese?
_____	_____	_____	_____
_____	_____	_____	_____
_____	_____	_____	_____

DEPRESSION OR ANXIETY

Who?	Current age?	Current health?	Obese?
_____	_____	_____	_____
_____	_____	_____	_____
_____	_____	_____	_____

OTHER

Who?	Current age?	Condition/Current health?	Obese?
_____	_____	_____	_____
_____	_____	_____	_____
_____	_____	_____	_____

For Your Spirit

Meditation

Being able to be still inside is an important aspect of making changes on the outside. Taking time to get quiet and centered within is an important part of your thirty-day *HealthQuest* program. One of the best ways to do this is through meditation.

Many people think meditation is only for people who practice Eastern religions. While it is an important part of some religions, meditation isn't just for aspiring yogis, and it doesn't conflict with any other religion.

You often hear meditation and prayer used interchangeably, but they're somewhat different. If you, like many Black folks, grew up in a traditional Black Christian church, you might make this analogy: Prayer is talking to God. Meditation is being still enough to listen.

The word "meditation" may conjure up images of people sitting cross-legged in white robes chanting mantras for hours. In fact, meditation is mostly about mind-set—the actual practice can take many different forms. There are people who do walking meditations, others who mediate while dancing, painting, flower arranging, making tea, or cooking. Know, too, that it can be a powerful and positive force for inner healing—and a calm, stress-free inner environment is one where physical healing can better take place as well.

When it comes to your diet, meditation gives you a way to deal with stress, nervousness, and the blues that's an alternative to eating. It lets you reach a deep state of relaxation, reduces tension, and helps you find your inner strength—the part of you that holds the power to make lasting life changes.

To meditate, you'll want to set aside twenty minutes, ideally at around the same time each day. You might find that you enjoy meditating first thing in the morning, or before your daily walk around the block, or after your evening meal. Whatever works for you.

Find a quiet place in your home where you won't be disturbed. Some folks set up an altar—it can be a bench or a small table—to indicate their meditation space. You can decorate it with candles, photos of dear relatives, flowers, seashells, or objects that reflect your spirituality or things you most deeply value. Or maybe your meditation place is by a window where you can look out on nature or up at the sky. The goal: a place that feels comfortable, pleasing, and peaceful.

[TIP: Some people—especially those who have children or who live with other people—say they find it difficult to find an uninterrupted space. Try meditating in the bathtub. It's quiet, you can close the door, and warm water is extra soothing.]

Sit comfortably on a pillow or chair and close your eyes. You want to come to a state of inner stillness. First, focus on breathing steadily in and out in a smooth, regular rhythm. You'll notice yourself relaxing. At first your mind may be racing—making to-do lists, remembering something that happened yesterday, wondering if this meditation is really going to work. Notice what that voice in your head is saying. You'll be tempted to try to stop it, to make it be still. But just notice your thoughts, then let them pass through your head. If you have difficulty letting go of thoughts, just tell yourself each time: "I can think about it later." Then set the thought aside. Just keep breathing slowly, deliberately, deeply, continuing to focus on just being right there in that moment—not the future, not the past.

With a little practice, you may become oblivious to everything around you, or feel as though you're detached from your body. That's the deep relaxation state you're after.

After about twenty minutes, open your eyes very slowly. If you're like most people, you'll feel refreshed, renewed, restored, and in closer touch with your inner self.

Meditation isn't hard, but frankly, it looks easier than it is. You may find it's easier to try it in small doses at first—just a few minutes at a time. That's fine. Your goal during your *HealthQuest* 30-Day Weight-Loss Program is to gradually work up to meditating for 20 minutes a day.

CHAPTER 7

Getting Down to Business

Defining Goals, Adopting Strategies, and Planning Meals

At this point you've identified some of your eating patterns and the types of foods you like to eat, have picked a food pyramid that feels best for you, and have determined your ideal weight and your weight-loss goals. Now it's time to get down to business. In this chapter, we'll get to the weight-loss process itself. Here we'll present two strategies for losing weight, one more rigorous than the other. You'll select the approach that seems best for you—although, of course, you're always free to change.

Once you've decided upon your weight-loss strategy, you'll analyze your food diary. Then we'll introduce you to a menu of techniques you can select from to replace your current high-fat, high-calorie menu with a healthier one. But don't feel intimidated; we're right here to help you. We'll introduce you to a two-week weight-loss menu containing delicious, low-calorie soul-food recipes. And we'll also teach you how to craft menu makeovers to fit your own taste and lifestyle, by using plenty of charts and helpful menu tips to make the whole process easier.

Lose Weight for Life

In the last chapter, you compared your actual weight with your ideal weight, so you should already have a good idea of how much weight you want to lose. Now you need a plan to make it happen. You need a strategy to lose weight.

But before we help you develop that strategy, let's talk seriously for a moment about the process of losing weight. As we told you earlier, the statistics on dieting can be sobering. Studies show that within two years, up to 90 percent of dieters will regain the weight they lost and some will gain even more weight. You can safely assume that many—perhaps, most—of the people in this 90 percent employed unhealthy weight-loss methods—some of the same gimmicks you may have tried yourself: diet pills, cabbage soup, high-protein diets, the soap that claims to melt fat. These methods cannot succeed when assessed against our sixteen-point criteria for a healthy weight-loss program.

Yet some people who lose weight succeed both in losing the weight and keeping it off. You know the ones—the people who go from fat to fit and fabulous, from chubby to curvaceous. Here are some facts that will help you increase the likelihood that you'll be in that exclusive club:

We think it's worth repeating that the best and, perhaps, only way to lose weight and keep it off for the long term is to approach weight-loss as a lifestyle change you will implement forever. People who successfully lose weight and keep it off give up living on autopilot; they plan their eating and exercising, and make weight loss and weight maintenance a conscious and intentional process. For example, rather than running out the door each morning without thinking about what they are going to eat that day, successful dieters may sit down the night before to plan their meals for the next day. Instead of following the lunchtime crowd to a fast-food restaurant, they may think carefully about whether that restaurant offers food choices compatible with their lifestyle. If not, they may choose to eat someplace else. They also make exercising a top priority and integrate it into their lives.

Most people who are successful at weight loss choose to lose very slowly—between one-half and two pounds per week, two to eight pounds per month. That means they don't set such aggressive objectives that they feel deprived of their favorite foods and, therefore, more likely to blow their diet on a late-night binge on a Mississippi mud pie. Nor do they make themselves overly uncomfortable by cutting their daily calorie intake so low that they're doubled over with hunger pains. In fact, studies show that you're mostly likely to succeed if your goal is to lose no more than 10 to 15 percent of your body weight. That's the equivalent of twenty to thirty pounds for a two-hundred-pound person, enough to see a change and experience the health-related benefits.

Our successful friends also focus on weight-loss maintenance. As a matter of fact, the National Institutes of Health suggests that after six months your primary goal should be to maintain the weight you've lost; any additional weight should be gravy. If you really accept the fact you're making lifestyle changes, maintaining your new weight shouldn't be too difficult. If you're successful, then start to move toward the weight the BMI says is best for you, if it's more than you've already lost.

If your objective is to lose weight quickly, we suggest that you plan to lose no more than eight pounds per month. Beyond that, it's considerably less likely that you'll be able to keep the weight off. So go easy on yourself. Eight pounds is a fantastic start, no matter what your ultimate weight-loss goal is.

"Yeah, right," you're saying. "But I want to lose one hundred pounds. At this pace, that'll take me a full year!"

You're right. If you're looking to lose more than a few pounds, it might seem like two to eight pounds a month is losing at a snail's pace. But wise weight loss, like anything done wisely, is a process that requires patience. You probably didn't put the weight on in a year, so be gentle with yourself and give yourself some time to take it off. Even if you're feeling motivated because you need to lose weight to alleviate a health condition, know that many health symptoms can be relieved by losing as little as ten to fifteen pounds. That can be accomplished safely in two to three months. (Be sure to ask your doctor if this is true for your ailment.) If you invest the time now in methodical weight removal, not only are you more likely to keep it off, you're less likely to experience the disappointment of failing. And you won't have to spend time and energy starting all over again.

For now don't even think about the total number of pounds you're trying to punt. Just concentrate on the weekly weight loss. As long as you're losing a pound or two each week, consider yourself a grand success. Before you know it, your weight loss will start adding up to significant figures—and a spectacular figure. Now we're going to help you develop a plan to get there from here.

Define Your Goal

Now that you know what it takes to succeed, let's take some time to fine-tune your weight-loss goals. Pull out your Food and Fitness Diary and write the answers to the following:

• Calculate 10 percent of your weight and write in that number. Most people who are successful at losing weight are able to lose at least this many pounds.

• Calculate 15 percent of your weight and write in that number. You are most likely to succeed if you lose no more than this many pounds.

• Write in the amount of weight you'd have to lose to reach the weight suggested by the Body Mass Index (BMI) chart on page 93.

• Calculate your ideal weight-loss goal and write that in.

To help you manage your expectations, let's calculate a range of months that you'll need to focus on weight loss.

• Calculate the so-called worst-case scenario by dividing your 15 percent weight-loss goal by two pounds per month. This tells you the maximum number of months you'll focus on weight loss, assuming you're losing two pounds per month. Write down that number.

• Calculate the best-case scenario by dividing your 10 percent weight-loss goal by eight pounds per month. This tells you the minimum number of months you'll focus on weight loss. It assumes you're losing at the maximum healthy weight-loss weight of eight pounds per month. Write down that number.

Now write a goal statement, breaking your weight-loss objective down into small, bite-sized nuggets. Something like:

My goal is to lose 30 pounds, the equivalent of 15 percent of my current weight of 200 pounds. I will enjoy shedding these pounds over the ten-

*month period between January and November of this year. That's the equiv-
alent of 3 pounds a month, less than a pound per week (actually, its 2,650
calories), about 375 calories a day.*

How to Cut Down the Pounds

N ow that you've set your weight-loss goals, it's time to focus on shedding the pounds. There are a couple of healthy ways to do it. By far
the most popular involves counting calories, paying attention both to the
number of calories you eat and the number you burn. A less common but
also effective weight-loss method is to nix counting calories and focus on
changing the proportion of foods on your plate, instead. Calorie-count-
ing, of course, is more rigorous. But both can be effective. First we'll talk
about counting calories, then we'll talk about reproportioning your plate.

How Calories Add Up

In chapter 3 you learned that calories are a measure of food energy, but
we more commonly think of them in terms of weight. When we wonder
how many calories are in that frosted cinnamon bun at the mall (more
than 600), it's because we want to know how much weight we'll gain if we
eat one. Now you already know that excess calories are stored on the body
as fat, but did you know that you need to eat only an extra 3,500 of them
and you'll pick up an additional pound? And wait till we show you how
easily that can happen.

Consider this common scenario: Say you treat yourself to one 100-
calorie chocolate chip cookie a day. That's an additional 3,000 calories in
a month, almost an entire pound. Add that up over the course of a year
and you've picked up about ten pounds. All from eating a little cookie.
That's not much wiggle—or jiggle—room.

On the flip-side, knowing that one cookie a day can result in so much
misery means that it may not be so difficult to lose weight after all.
Eliminate that same cookie from your daily diet and you *lose* a pound of
fat about every five weeks, about ten pounds a year. That's not so painful,
is it?

So let's break down this 3,500-calorie figure into more manageable
numbers. Thirty-five hundred calories is the equivalent of 500 calories

per day, seven days a week. If you want to lose a pound of fat a week, you'll have to eliminate about 500 calories a day. To lose a half a pound per week, you can cut that number in half; you'll only have to get rid of 1,500 calories a week, 250 a day. On the other hand, if you want to lose two pounds a week, you'll need to eliminate 7,000 calories, the equivalent of 1,000 calories per day.

But it's very difficult to eliminate 1,000 calories a day without feeling deprived. And depending upon how much you weigh, you may not even have 1,000 calories to spare. So we suggest that you choose to lose at a slower pace—say, one-half to one pound per week. That's only 250 to 500 calories per day.

How much sacrifice does that involve? Well, take a look at the list of processed foods below. We've listed processed foods because Americans tend to eat a lot of them, and as you learned earlier, they tend to be high in calories. Each item on this list contains between 220 and 250 calories, the equivalent of a light dinner consisting of a pork chop and a sweet potato. Eat two of these foods and chances are you've added an extra 500 calories that day. But eliminate two and you've cut 500 calories. You can do that, can't you?

APPROXIMATELY 220–250 CALORIES
2 handfuls of tortilla chips
1 ½ twelve-ounce cans or 1 twenty-ounce bottle of soda
5 saltines and 2 tablespoons of peanut butter
1 candy bar
2 one-inch cubes of cheese
4 tablespoons roasted almonds

Another way to approach it is to eliminate calories in small increments—a couple here and a couple there. This approach makes changing your diet less dramatic—and traumatic. You can still enjoy the foods you love; you just cut calories around the edges. For example, use skim milk on your cereal instead of whole milk and save 60 calories. Skip the mayo on your turkey sandwich and save 50 calories. Bake a chicken leg instead of frying it and save 85 calories. Take the skin off prior to eating it and save 45 more.

Easy enough, right? But, don't forget that exercise needs to play an important part in your weight-loss process. For reasons we'll discuss in chapter 8, you are much more likely to succeed if you incorporate more activity into your life. Ultimately, your objective will be to eliminate half of your daily calorie goal by changing food choices and the other half by burning them off by becoming more active. That means if your objective is to eliminate 500 calories a day, 250 will come from your diet and 250 from exercise. You are making a lifestyle change, not "dieting" remember? But for now, we'll just focus on changing your food choices.

Making Calories Count

It's important to know how many calories you need to cut, but you also need to know how many calories you can eat. You want to lose weight, not turn into a beanstalk. And there's no sense in cutting back so far that your colleagues at work can hear your stomach growling from three offices down the hall. On the other hand, you don't want to scarf down so many calories that cutting back will merely cause you to gain weight less quickly. You need to know how many calories a person your size can safely consume and still lose weight in a healthy manner.

According to dietitian Constance Brown-Riggs, by following a simple mathematical rule of thumb, you can calculate roughly how many calories you should eat, whether you want to lose, maintain, or gain weight. The mathematical formula reflects the fact that the human body will burn about twelve calories per pound just to maintain its current weight. Obviously, if you want to lose weight, you need to feed your body fewer calories than it requires for weight maintenance. The formulas apply whether you're male or female, but keep in mind the fact that they are approximate. You can do the calculation yourself—or if math wasn't your favorite subject, refer to the chart below.

Here's how the calculations work: To estimate how many calories you can eat and still lose weight, take your current weight and multiply it by 10. So, let's say you weigh 200 pounds. You should consume roughly 2,000 calories a day if you want to lose weight.

For weight maintenance, take your current weight and multiply it by 12. A 200-pound person who likes how much he or she weighs should eat 2,400 calories a day.

And in the unlikely event that someone you know wants to gain weight, tell them to multiply their current weight by 15. A 200-pound person who wants to pick up a couple of pounds should eat 3,000 calories a day.

Write your daily calorie goal in your Food and Fitness Diary.

One more important point about calorie consumption: Not only should you consume the number of calories recommended for your weight range, we suggest you consume a consistent number of calories every day. Don't starve yourself one day and binge the next. Your body will cop an attitude.

But what if I want to lose weight more rapidly than the rate you've recommended? While we discourage rapid weight loss, we do know that some of you will do it, anyway. If you insist, make sure to keep your daily calorie count within healthy limits. According to Brown-Riggs, most women can safely reduce their calorie intake to 1,200 to 1,500 calories per day, and men can go as low as 1,800 to 2,000 calories per day—but you shouldn't go below that. Remember that starving yourself and otherwise consuming too few calories can slow down your metabolism and actually prevent you from losing weight.

What does a 1,200-calorie day look like? Here's a healthy example. It's also a good starting point to build your daily diet upon. To increase the calorie count to bring it in line with your daily objective, identify foods

NUMBER OF CALORIES PER DAY			
Current Weight	Lose Weight	Maintain Weight	Gain Weight
125 lb.	1,250	1,500	1,875
150 lb.	1,500	1,800	2,250
175 lb.	1,750	2,100	2,625
200 lb.	2,000	2,400	3,000
225 lb.	2,250	2,700	3,375
250 lb.	2,500	3,000	3,750
275 lb.	2,750	3,300	4,125
300 lb.	3,000	3,600	4,500

you'd like to add and check their calorie count in appendix 1 on page 232, where you'll find nutritional information for an array of popular foods.

1,200 Calorie Sample Menu

Breakfast	Serving Size	Calories
Cornflakes	¾ cup	80
Banana	½ cup	60
Skim milk	½ cup	45
Totals:		185

Lunch	Serving Size	Calories
Whole wheat bread	2 slices	160
Lean roast beef	2 ounces	110
Tomato	1 large	25
Lettuce	2 leaves	0
Mayonnaise	1 teaspoon	45
Fresh peach	1 medium	60
Skim milk	½ cup	45
Totals:		445

Dinner	Serving Size	Calories
Roast loin pork	2 ounces	110
Brown gravy	2 tablespoons	80
Mashed potato	½ cup	80
Steamed collard greens	1 cup	50
Fresh strawberries	1 ¼ cups	60
Skim milk	½ cup	45
Margarine	1 teaspoon	45
Totals:		470

Snack	Serving Size	Calories
Ice cream, nonfat	½ cup	90

| Daily Calorie Total: | | 1,190 |

Do the Math

Now that you have an understanding of the number of calories you need to consume to lose weight, let's take another look at your week of eating in your food diary. Select a typical day—in fact, select a day when you were particularly "bad" in your eating, so you can really get the point. In your Food and Fitness Diary, make a chart similar to the one below; fill in the foods you ate on your selected day.

Now take the list to the kitchen and look at the nutrition labels of the foods you ate. Compare the amount you ate with the serving size on the label and multiply or divide in order to calculate the number of calories in each food item you consumed. For example, if the serving size listed on the bag of trail mix you munched on was a quarter cup and you chowed down on a half cup, you ate double the calories on the label. Jot down this calorie count beside each food you ate. (For things like meat or fresh vegetables that don't have a label, look at the chart in appendix 1.)

Next, sit down with the list and add up the numbers. In your Food and Fitness Diary, fill in your total calorie intake for the day. How does it compare to the number of calories you need to consume to maintain your weight? Lose weight? How many extra calories did you consume?

Food Item	Calories per Serving	Number of Servings	Total Calories
_____	_____	_____	_____
_____	_____	_____	_____
_____	_____	_____	_____
_____	_____	_____	_____
_____	_____	_____	_____
_____	_____	_____	_____
_____	_____	_____	_____
_____	_____	_____	_____
_____	_____	_____	_____
	Total Calories Consumed:		_____
	Daily Calorie Goal for Weight Loss:		_____
	Extra Calories Consumed:		_____

Look at the list again and mark items that you might have skipped to save yourself some calories. Keep marking items until you've eliminated 250 calories or have reached the daily calorie count you need to achieve to lose weight. Because junk foods and beverages contain so many calories, many people find that reducing or eliminating them is the easiest place to start. Try not to cut out nutritious vegetables and whole-grain foods. And perhaps you don't want to cut the whole dish, but cut your portion size instead—say, one sandwich instead of two. What's left is what your diet should look like if you want to eliminate 250 calories.

How does it look to you? Skimpy? Reasonable?

Do you think you could manage to live on that amount of food each day? If not, why?

What other kinds of adjustments could you make in your diet that would be more comfortable?

If you are surprised as you look at how much you eat, know that you are not alone. Many folks, overweight or not, have no idea how much they eat. Even a study of registered dietitians—people whose job it is to help others figure out how much to eat—found that they have the same problem. But between not being aware of how much we eat and not being aware of the number of calories found in our favorite foods, the calories creep in and pounds start to add up.

 Weight Gain and the Holiday Season

A recent study on holiday weight gain published in the *New England Journal of Medicine* tells an interesting story about how weight can accumulate slowly over our lifetime. Previous studies suggested that during adulthood, most Americans gain an average of 0.4 to 1.8 pounds per year. This study sought to determine how much of that weight gain occurs over the holidays.

The findings offer good news and bad news. The good news is that the average subject gained a little over a pound during the winter months, three-quarters of it between Thanksgiving and New Year's. That's less than the participants thought they gained. Participants who were more active gained less weight than those who were sedentary. (That's proof that burning calories works.) The bad news is that people who where already overweight or obese were more likely to gain *five* pounds during the holiday season.

Not surprisingly, most of the study participants didn't lose their winter weight when the weather warmed up; they weighed in about 1.5 pounds heavier the next year. The "cumulative effects of yearly weight gain during the fall and winter are likely to contribute to the substantial increase in body weight that frequently occurs during adulthood," the study reported. That is to say, the weight gained during the holidays is unlikely to come off.

Think about it. If you pick up 1.5 pounds per year between ages twenty-one and forty-one, that's a total of thirty pounds. By age fifty-one, you'll weigh forty-five pounds more than in your early twenties; by age sixty-one, you'll weigh sixty pounds more. And the weight accumulates one bite at a time, much of it during the holiday season.

This begs the question of how to develop a strategy to deal with the holidays. We're going to help you develop one here by using typical holiday fare as our starting point for examining food choices.

Here's a typical holiday dinner and a lower-calorie counterpart. Compare the two meals and the respective calorie counts. You can see how easy it is to pack on weight and how, by modifying your diet, you can still enjoy the same fantastic flavors without being penalized in the form of fat.

Traditional Holiday Meal		Modified Holiday Meal	
Food	**Calories**	**Food**	**Calories**
Appetizer			
¼ cup assorted nuts	349	1 cup fruit cup	245
2 oz. potato chips	278		
Dinner			
4 oz. turkey, light and dark meat	176	3 oz. white turkey	94
½ cup cranberry sauce	208	¼ cup cornbread stuffing	90

1 cup cornbread stuffing	356	¼ cup defatted gravy	22
¼ cup gravy	164	4 oz. baked sweet potato	117
½ cup mashed potatoes	111	½ cup collard greens (no fat)	15
½ cup collard greens	64	½ cup carrots	35
½ cup buttered corn	125	½ cup broccoli	22
½ cup candied yams	101	1 cup wine spritzer	80
2 oz. cornbread	179		
2 cups white wine	321		

Dessert

1 slice sweet potato pie	316	1 slice sweet potato pie	316
¼ cup vanilla ice cream	90		

Night Snack

1 turkey sandwich	252	No night-time snack	0

Total Calories	**3,090**	**Total Calories**	**1,034**

What does all this mean? Well, if a 150-pound woman were to eat the traditional, down-home holiday meal instead of sticking to her weight-loss target of 1,500 calories, she would consume 3,090 calories in a single sitting. That's over twice her daily goal—not including what she ate for breakfast and lunch—and almost an extra half a pound. If she eats either breakfast or lunch, we can reasonably assume that this sister would gain at least a half pound on that one day alone, mostly from losing control on a single meal.

But if our same 150-pound woman were willing to control her portion sizes and make a few meal substitutions, she could still enjoy the same flavors she loves, stay within her weight-loss objective of 1,500 calories a day, and still have 500 calories left over for breakfast and lunch. Even if she decided to treat herself to some extra servings of stuffing, she could easily stay below the 1,800-calorie total she could safely consume that day to maintain her weight.

Now imagine these two scenarios playing out several times during the holiday season. Our sister-friend may not know it, but she's at a fork in the road. If she takes one path, she could easily gain five pounds or more come New Year's Day; if she takes the other, she could weigh five pounds less. That's a ten-pound spread in only a six-week period of time!

This is a dramatic example of just how dramatic small changes can be as they accumulate over time—and of how deadly the holidays can be if you don't have a plan to manage your food choices. Counting calories is a good place to start; every choice to save calories adds up. In a short period of time, you can lose a good amount of weight. But there are other strategies you might find more comfortable and easy to manage. Create an approach that's right for you.

Reproportion Your Plate

Easier than counting calories, and perhaps as effective, is changing the proportions of foods on your plate. Instead of making meat the center of your meal, reduce your fat and protein servings to one-third of your plate (remember, animal protein contains saturated fat and cholesterol), and fill the other two-thirds with fruits, vegetables, and grains (carbohydrates). Believe it or not, by making this simple change, you can make a tremendous impact on your weight without counting calories. Assuming you don't select too many foods that are highly processed, changing your plate proportions should cut your calories way down and give you incredible health benefits.

But just because you choose to change the proportions of foods on your plate doesn't mean that you can't also benefit from other methods to reduce calories and improve your health.

BEFORE	AFTER

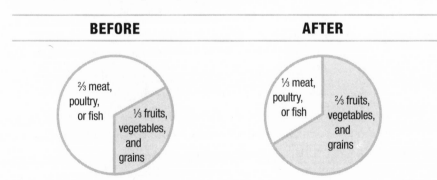

⅔ meat, poultry, or fish ⅓ fruits, vegetables, and grains

⅓ meat, poultry, or fish ⅔ fruits, vegetables, and grains

Eight Ways to Cut Calories from Your Diet

Y ou've made it. After all this reading, you've finally arrived at the part of the book where we help you develop your strategy to save calories—one that's active on all fronts, at home and away, whether you're in front of the pantry, menu, or the frozen-food section. These are the easiest and most effective places to find extra calories to eliminate from your diet. Remember, you're looking for ways to trim a couple of calories here, a couple there. All totaled, they should add up to the number of calories you plan to eliminate from your diet each day.

1. Reduce Calories from Beverages

Next time you leave your work station to buy a drink from the vending machine, you might want to consider hitting the water cooler, instead. Most of us don't think about the number of calories beverages add to our daily diets, but the calorie count is rising rapidly. More and more of us are consuming juice, sodas, teas, and flavored waters instead of that old standby, water. According to the U.S. Department of Agriculture, the average American adult now drinks about forty gallons of sweetened soda pop per year, up from about twenty-two gallons in 1970. Assuming there are about 10 calories in an ounce of soda, that's the equivalent of over seven pounds of excess calories consumed in pop alone. Each year. And that's just sweetened soda. We didn't include fruit juice, tea, flavored waters, or any other calorie-containing beverage.

"Beverages are a huge contributor to obesity," says Richard Mattes, Ph.D., professor of nutrition at Purdue University, in the *Nutrition Action Newsletter*, a publication of the Center for Science in the Public Interest. "Over the last twenty years, we've gotten fatter, but what's really changed is that we're drinking a lot more calories than we ever did before."

Part of the reason is because serving sizes are ballooning. There was a time when pop was served in 12-ounce cans (and depending how old you are, you may remember 8-ounce sizes). Now, a single serving is more likely to be a 20-ounce bottle, with 32-ounce drinks frequently marketed to young people. Sodas are even served in 64-ounce cups at some convenience stores and movie theaters. That's an increase from around 120 calories for a 12-ounce can, to 310 calories for a 32-ounce drink, up to 600 calories for a 64-ounce cup. It's easy to see how a couple of sodas a day can take up a significant portion of your daily calorie count. This upsizing of beverages has the most significant consequences for men, who are the objects of the large drink advertising. A man who consumes 64 ounces of soda a day is likely to be consuming a quarter of his daily calories from beverages alone. Worse, he'll still find himself feeling hungry.

Why? Your body isn't satisfied by liquid calories the way it is by food calories. As a result beverages often contribute "stealth" calories—liquids enter our body, but unlike when we eat foods, the mechanism that tells us when we're full is unable to detect them.

"Liquid calories don't trip our satiety mechanisms," said Dr. Mattes. "They don't even register."

So how do you circumvent this problem? One obvious answer is to drink more water and less soda and fruit juices. Remember, your body needs at least 64 ounces of water per day but most of us don't consume that much. You can also reduce the size of drink you order, switch to diet drinks, and dilute juices with water or seltzer.

Note the food label on the beverages you drink and the number of calories they contain. Keep this in mind as you consider your beverage choices.

2. Reduce Serving Sizes

In chapter 4 we told you how important it is to understand proper serving sizes. Let's review them by returning to page 74 and reminding ourselves of the suggested serving sizes for each food group, since they're a lot different from what most of us are used to eating. We encourage you to be patient with yourself as you overcome your old habits, but eating proper serving sizes will have a visible impact on your weight. Sometimes this is easier said than done, but here are a few tips to make the transition easier.

When you're at home, you have complete control over serving sizes. So you'll need to practice mindfulness and discipline when filling up your plate and dishing out snacks. To reduce the temptation to eat supersize servings, we suggest breaking down large bags of snack items—whether potato chips or grapes—into smaller sandwich bags that reflect healthy portion sizes. That way, you define the serving size when you're not hungry and are more likely to follow the pyramids. Then when you want a snack, the serving size is predefined, so you're less likely to overeat. This approach is a great way to prevent yourself from overeating processed foods.

Eating in a restaurant is another story. Because you're not in control, you've really got to be on guard, especially because it's becoming more common for restaurants to serve oversize portions. We'll give you more tips on eating out later in this chapter. For now, the best way to protect yourself is to ask that the dish be split in the kitchen and ask the chef or waiter to put half in a doggie bag and delivered with your check. Now you can savor the wonderful presentation, the fragrances and flavors of your food, and the fact that someone else did all the work, without worrying that you'll overeat. If you're in a fast-food restaurant, best to just order the smallest sizes of every food, whether a hamburger, fries, or a shake.

3. Eat Healthier Foods

One of the easiest ways to lose weight is to incorporate more healthy foods into your diet. As you learned earlier, diets containing a cornucopia of fruits, vegetables, and other plant-based foods are naturally low in fat and calories. That's why our second weight-loss strategy doesn't require that you count calories but merely alter the proportions of food on your plate to increase the number of carbohydrates. As you compare the calorie count of the following foods, notice the difference in calorie count between processed and unprocessed carbs:

Processed and Unprocessed Foods

FOOD	SERVING SIZE	CALORIES
Baked potato	1 medium	88
Biscuit	1	276
Broccoli	1 cup	25
Cornbread	1 slice	179
French fries	20–25	250
Grapes	1 cup	101

Grits, hominy	1 cup	145
Pasta with cheese and sauce	1 cup	300
Peach cobbler	⅛ pie	300
Pizza, deluxe	1 slice	309
Pot pie	1	395
Rice, white	1 cup	267
Watermelon	1 cup	48

Another way to reduce the calories in the foods you eat is to alter the ingredients to make them more healthy. If you find yourself eating a lot of high-fat, high-calorie foods, try substituting these lower-calorie ingredients instead:

Substitutions List

Instead of:	Substitute:
Whole milk	Skim or 1% milk
Evaporated milk	Evaporated skim milk
Light cream	Equal amounts of 1% milk and evaporated skim milk
Heavy cream	Evaporated skim milk
1 cup butter	1 cup soft margarine or ⅔ cup vegetable oil*
Oil, butter, or margarine in baked goods	An equal amount of applesauce. If oil is the only liquid, substitute a mixture of applesauce and buttermilk instead.
Shortening or lard	Soft margarine*
Mayonnaise or salad dressing	Nonfat or light mayonnaise or salad dressing; use mustard in sandwiches
Eggs	¼ cup egg substitute or 2 egg whites
Cheese	Lower fat cheese**
Cream cheese	Nonfat or light cream cheese
Sour cream	Nonfat or low-fat sour cream or yogurt
Fat for greasing pan	Nonstick cooking spray

1 ounce baking chocolate	3 tablespoons cocoa powder plus 1 tablespoon vegetable oil
Chocolate	An equal amount of prune puree or prune baby food
Frosting	Replace butter or margarine with marshmallow cream
Regular bouillon or broth	Low-sodium bouillon or broth
Fatback, neck bone, or ham hocks	Skinless chicken thighs
Pork bacon	Turkey bacon, lean ham or Canadian bacon (omit if on low-sodium diet)
Pork sausage	Turkey breast
Ground beef and pork	Ground skinless turkey breast

* The texture of baked goods may be different when you use these substitutions. "Light" margarine is not recommended for baking. Experiment to find out what works best for you.

** Some salad dressings, processed cheeses, and cottage cheese are very high in sodium. Omit if on a low-sodium diet or substitute a product that is low in sodium and fat.

4. Snack Smart

Grazing can be good. That is, eating a little bit every couple of hours instead of waiting to eat the big three meals each day. "This helps to keep the metabolism revved up and hunger pangs down," says our nutrition expert Constance Brown-Riggs. But take it from the cows, grazing doesn't mean a can of soda, cheese and crackers, microwave popcorn, a candy bar, potato chips, tortilla chips, cheese puffs, and the rest of what you're likely to find in the snack machine at work. Eat a lot of these types of food and they're likely to take up residence around our waistlines.

Still, who doesn't love a slice of lemon pound cake or a bag of Cheez Doodles or cookies and ice cream every now and then? Isn't it possible to eat the snack foods we love without feeling guilty about it? The answer to that question is *Yes*—in moderation. It's important that you understand that there are no good or bad foods. Sounds so nice, we'll say it twice: *There are no good or bad foods.* Hallelujah! Having said that, however, there are foods that are healthier for us than others, as well as foods that we only want to savor in small amounts.

What kinds of foods are we talking about? Well, it won't surprise you that the ones we want to enjoy in small amounts are the ones at the top of the food pyramid. And even though some of those foods are available in low-fat versions, you should still eat them sparingly. Remember, highly processed foods tend to be high in calories and low in nutrition—even the low-fat ones.

Wait a minute! you're saying. *I thought I was doing a good thing by buying low-fat cookies; now you're trying to tell me that they'll make me gain weight, too?* Well, not exactly, but there are some important facts you need to know about low-fat treats.

We've been led to believe that by substituting low-fat snacks for their full-fat counterparts, we can literally have our cake and eat it, too; we can continue to enjoy our favorite goodies without having to pay the price by getting fat. But the misconception that these foods leave may actually set you up to gain more weight.

Take low-fat baked goods. Perhaps you've scarfed down more low-fat cookies than you ordinarily would have because you thought there'd be no negative consequences. If so, you're not alone—but you are misinformed. The fact that these foods are low in fat doesn't mean they're low in calories. That's news to you, right? So go see for yourself. Head into the kitchen and take a look at the nutrition facts label on your favorite low-fat cookies or ice cream. First check out the calorie count, then look at the serving size. Shocking, huh?

Many low-fat sweets contain a lot of calories because they contain a lot of sugar. And you already know that excess calories, whether from fat, carbohydrates (remember, sugar is a carb), or any other type of food will cause you to gain weight. So while eating low-fat snack foods can help, it doesn't negate the fact that you're still consuming calories.

In fact, food experts describe many of our favorite snack foods as being *calorie dense*. That's a sophisticated way of saying they have a lot of calories in each bite. But the concept is important because the more calories are in each bite of food you eat, the more total calories you're likely to eat.

Think of the difference between a bite of spinach, for instance, and a bite of premium cheesecake. Spinach has about 6 calories per ounce, while premium cheesecake has about 99. An apple has about 17 calories per ounce; broiled flounder, about 34; grilled chicken, about 43; and a tuna salad sandwich, about 65. But check out these common highly processed snack items. While premium low-fat ice cream has only about 51 calories per ounce, that's over three times as many as you'll get in a bite of apple. Cheese nachos have about 113 calories per ounce; a chocolate bar, about 150; and butter or margarine, about 204. Wow, what a difference in the amount of fat contained in processed and unprocessed foods!

So we suggest you snack on your favorite fruits and veggies, instead. We know, we know—celery sticks are not as much fun as fried mozzarella sticks. But if you don't savor the flavor of cauliflower florets, try succulent strawberries, wonderful watermelon, red and green peppers, peaches that drip down your chin, or tart Granny Smith apples instead. Be patient with yourself; after a while, your tastes will begin to change. Soon you'll love the crispy crunch of celery between your teeth and the chewiness of its fiber. If you have a taste for fat, satisfy it by dipping your celery in a small amount of peanut butter or combining it with a small piece of low-fat cheese. You can do the same with apple slices. The good news is, you don't need to eliminate fried mozzarella sticks from your diet. Just follow the advice of the food guide pyramid: Eat fats, sweets, and processed foods sparingly.

Here's another piece of good news about incorporating unrefined carbohydrates into your diet. Today, you can reduce the amount of preparation time by buying ready-to-eat vegetables, like peeled baby carrots or precut celery sticks.

Still, we know there will be times when you'll want to eat ice cream and cookies or other processed foods. If you choose to indulge, we do recommend that you eat the low-fat version, just do so in moderation. The low-fat version of premium ice cream can contain 200 calories less than the full-fat version of the same brand. And Canadian- or turkey bacon, both of which are lower in fat than pork bacon, also contain less than half the calories. But don't forget to follow the advice of the food pyramid in terms of serving sizes and the number and size of daily portions.

Another strategy for success is to reduce the variety of snacks you bring into the house. Say you decide to get three bags of potato chips for your household. Instead of buying one bag of regular, one bag of barbecue, and one bag of sour cream and onion, purchase three bags of only one flavor. Studies show that there's no way you'll eat as much; you—and your family—will get sick of them first.

Finally, when you're snacking, don't walk around nibbling; sit down and eat, instead. Sitting down at the table will focus your attention and you're less likely to engage in unconscious eating. Same as when you're eating a meal.

5. Develop Restaurant Savvy

"But what about when I'm not preparing my own food," you ask. *"I can brown bag it from time to time, but I usually eat lunch in the cafeteria at work. I like to go out to brunch with my husband on Sundays, and I'll be eating at a wedding reception this weekend."*

Glad you asked! Because restaurant meals of any type are usually higher in calories than meals eaten at home (a single restaurant meal can easily contribute more than 1,000 calories to your daily calorie count), you're going to need a strategy for eating out. Don't worry; we've got you covered. When you're not in charge of the kitchen, you may have less control over your options, but you always have some control over what's served or how you handle what's set before you. Try following some of these suggestions so you can focus on enjoying your food and the friends who surround you:

• Whenever possible, and it often is possible, select a restaurant with a menu that supports your healthy, low-calorie eating habits. You can always look at the menu before you sit down, so that way you don't have to deal with the discomfort of getting up and leaving. Many restaurants display their menu in the window or lobby.

• If you have to go someplace where you know the menu isn't going to be prepared with the slightest nod to good health, then make sure you drink lots of water and eat a healthy minimeal before you go. That way you can say, "No thanks, I'm not very hungry"—and mean it.

• Ask to be seated away from the buffet table, the salad bar, the kitchen, and any areas where you can watch the food being prepared and the primary routes for bringing food from the kitchen into the dining room. No need to be drooling over other people's food all night.

• Let the waiter know that you're trying to lose weight. He can steer you to lower-calorie menu items.

• Assert yourself and make your needs known. Tell the waitress that you need her help selecting a low-calorie meal. Ask how the food is prepared and what's in it. If you don't like what you see, ask if the chef would be willing to prepare a special, low-calorie dish for you.

• Many restaurants offer a variety of choices that are lower in fat and calories. Look for those items on the menu. Sometimes they have a special "heart healthy" or "low fat" designation. Items listed as "vegetarian" may also be lower in fat or calories, but we don't guarantee it.

• Steer clear of items containing these descriptions: au gratin, buttery, casserole, creamed, creamy, crispy, fried, gravy, prime, scalloped, stewed. Their calories really add up.

• Don't order from an all-you-can-eat buffet. You'll tend to overeat.

• Have the bread, tortilla chips, and snack items removed from the table. Remember how quickly snack calories can add up? If you're in an upscale restaurant, hand back the wine menu and ask them not to bring the dessert cart to the table.

• Skip the appetizer. Many of the most popular appetizer items, like fried shrimp, fried Buffalo wings, mozzarella sticks, and egg rolls are high in calories and saturated fat. Just look at the menu and count the number of appetizers that are battered and fried.

• Order an appetizer- or lunch-sized portion for your main meal. Many restaurants are willing to serve you smaller portions than appear on the entrée portion of the menu. You only have to ask. Lunch portions are usually half the size of the dinner menu.

- Order your sauces, dressings, and butter on the side. That way you stay in control of what's on your plate.

- Trim the fat. When the plate is put before you, assess what you can do to avoid some of the calories staring at you. Can you trim some fat from the meat or take the skin off your chicken? Push the piece of ham hock away from your string beans and move the heavy dressing off your lettuce leaves. Blot the grease off your piece of pizza. Then resolve to eat only a healthy-sized portion. (Remember to use the portion size guidelines on page 74 as your rule of thumb.)

- Use a doggie bag. Many restaurants serve twice as much food as is healthy for you to eat. As we suggested earlier, ask your server to have the chef serve half and doggie-bag the rest. That way you won't be tempted to eat everything on your plate—or end up doing so unconsciously.

You can even order a healthy meal on an airplane. A wide variety of special meals are often available, ranging from vegetarian, vegan, and lacto-ovo vegetarian to lactose-free to kosher to fresh fruit and vegetable plates and even cold seafood. Not only are these meals tasty, they are prepared last, so their ingredients are usually fresher than those of a standard airplane meal. It's as simple as calling the airline twenty-four hours in advance and telling them what you want.

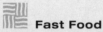 **Fast Food**

A large order of fries, a bacon burger with cheese on it, a nine-piece order of chicken nuggets. All of these foods taste great and they're definitely ready in a jiffy, but relying on fast food as a source of meals can really cause you to pack on pounds. Here's how:

A 150-pound woman trying to maintain her weight should eat about 1,800 calories a day. But by eating a typical lunch at the local burger joint—an order of small fries, a quarter-pound hamburger with cheese, and a large soda—she's stacking the deck against herself. In that one meal, she may easily consume

1,200 calories. And that may not be her largest meal. If she supersizes her meal, her calorie count may go off the chart.

To make matters worse, fast food is also high in saturated fat, sodium, and cholesterol. So what should you eat when you go to a fast-food restaurant?

Order the smallest burger available and ask for it to be cooked well done. The longer it cooks, the less fat it contains.

Avoid fried chicken or fried chicken sandwiches; they can have more calories than a hamburger. Order grilled or roasted skinless chicken, or skinless chicken sandwiches, or grilled or broiled fish, or fish sandwiches instead.

Check out the wraps or pita sandwiches. They're a great low-calorie alternative, as long as the meat is low fat (try chicken). Be sure to order low-calorie toppings, like lettuce, tomatoes, and onions. And watch out for high-calorie dressings.

Order the smallest order of fries available. Even then, dump a couple in the trash on your way to your table. If you order a stuffed potato, ask for it to be prepared without butter; order fat-free versions of cheese or sour cream, instead.

Order toppings carefully. Bacon and cheese each add around 100 calories to your sandwich. Order mustard instead of mayonnaise and save around 85 calories. Other low-fat dressings include salsa, barbecue sauce, and fat-free salad dressings.

6. Use Healthy Cooking Methods

In addition to making healthy food choices, we need to prepare food in a way that doesn't undermine all our effort. A nice fillet of trout is a healthy, low-calorie choice as long as you don't deep-fry it. A vegetable stir-fry can be a healthy, low-calorie meal—but not if it's dripping with oil and drowning in salty soy sauce. We may give ourselves a pat on the back for eating more broccoli, but if we smother it in cheese sauce we negate all our hard work. So in addition to counting calories in your food, you have to take into consideration how you're going to prepare it.

How you cook your food can make a world of difference in its calorie count and nutritional value. In chapter 3 we told you about the dangers of eating too much fat. Because excess fat can be so dangerous—espe-

Cooking Methods

Method	Pros	Cons
Roasting Cooking food uncovered in an oven with no moisture added. Use a rack to allow fat to drip off.	Roasting retains nutrients and flavor. Low oven temp (300–350) increases the amount of fat that drips off.	High oven temp (above 350) sears the meat and seals in the fat.
Baking Cooking food in an oven, covered.	Ideal for less fatty meats, retains moisture and blends flavors. Vegetables baked in their skins retain nutrients better than boiling.	Not good for less tender cuts of meat.
Broiling/Grilling Cooking by direct heat, either over or under the heat source. When using a gas range, keep oven door closed; when using an electric range crack the oven door slightly to prevent moisture from building up and slowing the browning process.	Great for reducing fat calories as fat drips away.	You need a rack to hold the meat out of the fat, and to keep the meat from stewing in its own juices and burning the fat.
Pan broiling Meat is placed in a heavy skillet with no added fat or water. Fat is removed as it accumulates.	Reduce fat calories by pouring off fat as it accumulates.	Pour off fat as it accumulates to prevent frying the meat in its own fat.
Frying Cooking food in small amounts of fat or deep-frying by submerging food in fat and cooking until crisp.	We do have to admit that frying's quick and the fat tastes good.	Usually involves batters, which increase the absorption of fat. Many people don't heat the oil properly, thereby increasing fat absorption.

Sautéing/Stir-Frying

Frying food quickly over a moderately high temp in a little fat. Requires frequent turning. Stir-frying is similar to sautéing with foods moved quickly in very little fat.

Retains flavor and nutrients of vegetables. You use less fat than regular or deep-frying methods.

Some calories are added from fat. Vegetables can be sautéed in broth to reduce fat.

Steaming/Pressure-Cooking

Cooking by contact with steam in a covered pot or perforated basket placed over hot water. Pressure-cooking is steaming under pressure.

Shortens cooking time for less tender cuts of meat. Water-soluble vitamins and flavor are retained in vegetables.

Vegetables take longer to cook than boiling.

Boiling/Poaching

Food is submerged into boiling water or broth and cooked thoroughly. (Meats are usually not boiled.) Poaching is cooking in a simmering liquid just below the boiling point.

Shortens cooking time for vegetables.

You lose more water, soluble vitamins, and flavor because vegetables are submerged in liquid.

Braising

Browning meat or vegetables first in fat, then slowly cooking in small amounts of liquid or sauce in a covered pan.

Tenderizes tough cuts of meat.

Fat remains in the cooking liquid and adds calories.

Microwave

Microwaves are absorbed by the food, causing water molecules to vibrate rapidly. The friction produces heat, which cooks the food.

Good for reheating cooked meats. You get less of that left-over flavor than reheating in a conventional oven.

Not good for large cuts of meat; it leaves some parts undercooked and others overcooked.

cially for African-Americans—we suggest you develop a healthy fear of frying.

Say, whaaaaaat! That can of bacon grease has been sitting next to your stove for three generations. And you've had lard in your cupboard for so long, you probably wouldn't know what to do without it. But it's time to give them the old heave-ho, and you can throw the deep fryer right on out with them! It's a new day. You live in a new millennium. If that doesn't help, the knowledge that you're holding on to a remnant from slavery should make you apoplectic. As we told you in the introduction, frying is a cultural retention from an era of night-riders and nursemaids, Bull Connors and bullwhips. So you owe it to the race to send the fat packing. It's time to broaden your kitchen skills and explore some healthier ways to cook.

What do we have in mind? Low- and no-fat cooking methods, like baking, broiling, grilling, poaching, microwaving, steaming, and stir-frying are all healthier alternatives. Check out the pros and cons of these cooking methods.

As much as we may love and be accustomed to the flavor of fried foods, low-fat and no-fat cooking methods can produce equally flavorful foods—once you know how to work them. These suggestions will help you cut the fat:

- Get yourself a good set of no-stick skillets, saucepans, and baking pans so you can sauté, fry, stir-fry, and bake without adding much fat, if any at all.

- Try sautéing vegetables in water, one to two tablespoons of defatted or low-sodium chicken or beef broth, juice, or wine.

- Replace full-fat cheeses with low-fat versions, but finely shred low-fat cheese because it doesn't melt as smoothly. Don't use fat-free cheeses on pizzas, casseroles, or sandwiches; use reduced-fat cheese instead.

- Cut any visible fat from meats before preparing them.

- Remove the skin before cooking poultry. Or, to keep the meat moist, leave the skin on during cooking, but remove it before eating. Studies show that the fat from the skin doesn't penetrate the meat during cooking. Of course, you'll have to apply seasonings under the skin if you want the meat to pick up their flavor.

• When you make soup at home, skim the fat before serving. One way to do this is to chill it and allow the fat to harden before you skim it off.

• Cut the fat in places it won't be missed, but keep the flavor of fatty ingredients like bacon, chocolate, coconut, and nuts by reducing the amount you use in recipes by 25 to 50 percent.

• You can often reduce the sugar in baked goods by as much as 25 percent, although sometimes reducing the sugar can affect the texture or volume of the item.

7. Spice Up Your Life

And while we're on the subject of trying new things, when you're learning new ways to cook, it's also a great time to experiment with new foods, ingredients, and flavors. Healthy meals should contain a lot of variety. By eating a wide variety of fruits, vegetables, grains, and other foods, we help ensure that we take in the full spectrum of vitamins and minerals that our bodies need each day. But not only do most of us tend to eat the same things over and over in a tight rotation, we often stick to the types of food we've always eaten instead of branching out and expanding our palettes.

But as our nation becomes more ethnically diverse, we have the opportunity to be exposed to new types of ethnic foods. Many of these foods are very tasty and contain healthy ingredients. In every major city—and many smaller ones—there are restaurants, supermarkets, and health-food stores that carry foods and ingredients from Asia and Southeast Asia, India, South and Central America, and the Caribbean. These can be excellent places to look for something unconventional (but healthy) for dinner.

Try eating out at more ethnic restaurants. Inquire about the flavors and ingredients you enjoy the most. Then scoop up a new cookbook, head to the ethnic food aisle in your supermarket (or, better, spice up your life by heading to a real ethnic market), and start to try them at home. The more diversity you have in your diet, the less likely you are to get bored and run for the cookie jar to satisfy your need for something different.

Even if you're not ready to turn into an ethnic epicurean, you can still make the low-calorie versions of your old favorites taste great. (We know you're trying to cook more healthily, but would never sacrifice your reputation for throwin' down.) Try experimenting with herbs and spices. They can zest up your food while keeping the calories down, especially when you want to replace fat or salty or sugary flavors.

These days you can get both fresh and dried herbs in most supermarkets (or have fun and grow them at home!). Dried herbs are located in the spice section and fresh ones can usually be found with produce. If you decide to experiment with fresh herbs, know that you use them differently than the dried ones you may be used to cooking with. Fresh herbs are less potent and their delicate taste tends to diminish the longer you cook them, so you'll want to add them at the end of the recipe, whereas dried herbs can cook right along with the other ingredients. And if you need to substitute dry herbs for fresh ones, use only one-third of what the recipe calls for. Try experimenting with these tasty combinations:

Fruit: cinnamon, cloves, ginger, mint
Vegetables: basil, chives, dill, parsley
Soups: bay leaves, marjoram, rosemary, tarragon
Poultry: garlic, oregano, rosemary, sage
Fish: chervil, dill, tarragon, thyme
Beef: chives, cumin, garlic, rosemary
Pork: black or cayenne pepper, garlic, rosemary, thyme

8. Eat at the Table, Not in Front of the TV

Finally, if there's one thing that's clear about Americans' eating habits, it's the fact that the TV encourages bad ones. Not only are poor eating habits reinforced on TV, when we eat in front of it, we numb out, become less mindful of how much we eat, and don't even savor food's wonderful flavors.

We suggest you turn off the TV whenever you eat, no matter whether you're enjoying a snack, a beverage, or a meal. Sit at the table so you can focus on your family's food culture, not the values and culture displayed on television.

So take a break from TV time. Enjoy preparing your food, inhale the fragrant aromas as you cook, be creative in your presentation, enjoy the wonderful colors, and flavors as you take in its nourishment. If you want, set the table, turn down the lights, light some candles, and listen to some mood music. But whatever you do, turn off the idiot box.

Planning Healthy Meals

By now you have a better sense of what a calorie-conscious menu looks like, so it's time to start applying that knowledge to your own actual menu and shopping lists. There are three ways to do this: (1) follow the *HealthQuest* Two-Week Menu Plan provided in appendix 2; (2) create your own healthy, low-calorie menus; (3) combine your healthy menu items with some of the delicious, low-fat, low-calorie recipes provided in appendix 3.

The *HealthQuest* Two-Week Menu Plan

If you want to start changing your diet but don't want to be burdened by counting calories, follow our two-week breakfast, lunch, and dinner menus. These menus are low in fat and calories, and provide you with proper nutrition and variety. The total calorie count for each day is about 1,200. The menus begin on page 252 in appendix 2. Here's an example of a typical 1,200-calorie day:

BREAKFAST
½ cup cooked oatmeal
2 tbsp. raisins
1 cup light soy milk
1 tsp. margarine
Calorie-free beverage

LUNCH

2 slices whole-wheat bread

2 oz. lean fresh ham

1 cup raw carrot sticks

1 small apple

2 tsp. russian dressing

Calorie-free beverage

DINNER

2 oz. JERK CHICKEN

1 cup CARIBBEAN RICE AND PEAS

2 cups tossed salad

2 tbsp. vinaigrette salad dressing

1 small orange

Calorie-free beverage

SNACK

1 cup soy vanilla yogurt

Calorie-free beverage

If your weight-loss objectives call for more calories than that, we suggest you look over appendix 1 and use the nutritional information chart to identify the calorie count for the items you'd like to add to the daily menu. Be sure to add items in proportions that reflect the advice of the food pyramids.

Create Your Own Healthy Menu

Another way to approach your dietary changes is to develop your own healthy menus based on the foods you and your family prefer to eat. Developing your own menu can be more work, but it allows you more control of the foods you eat.

Use your Food and Fitness Diary to plan a menu for the week. But before you start, grab your calendar and note things like luncheons, parties, meetings, and other occasions that might cause you to eat off schedule, in restaurants or otherwise, and tempt you to go off your weight-loss program. Leave a blank space for those meals.

Just go from the hip, right now—don't count calories or do any calculations. As much as possible, try to create a menu that's close to what you and your family normally eat. You can adjust later—but do it based on what your current eating style is, rather than introducing a whole new (read: foreign) menu. No need to fix what's not broken. And we find that, in most cases, we can find ways to substitute what you're currently eating with substitutions so close that you won't miss the real thing. More on that later.

Weekly menu done? Now count the calories for every meal. If you find that your menu includes more calories than your daily calorie goal, begin to look for places to cut. Don't forget to use the calorie lists in appendix 1 and the ingredients-substitutions list given earlier (on page 118) to help you quickly identify healthier replacements for some common ingredients. You can also use the *HealthQuest* meal-substitution list that follows to help you make better choices for some of the common foods that you enjoy. You'll find the calorie counts for these foods in the appendix, as well.

And don't forget to compare your daily menus with the food pyramids in chapter 4. If you need to add a few more vegetables, fruits, or grains—and most of us could afford to—or cut a serving or two of meat or fatty foods, now's the time to do it. Adjust the menu until it comes into the correct calorie range.

HealthQuest Meal-Substitutions

Combine Menus

The third option is to combine items from the *HealthQuest* Two-Week Menu Plan with items from your own menu. This option combines the familiarity of eating your own recipes with the flexibility to substitute a preplanned meal when needed. Don't forget to select menu items or recipes with an eye to your calorie count for the day. And always use the food pyramid to guide your food choices.

If all this thinking about menus seems like a lot of work, just realize that it'll get easier the more you do it. At some point it will become second nature. That's what you want, ultimately: for this kind of menu planning

Typical Choice	*HealthQuest* Choice
Breakfast	
Eggs, bacon, and cheese on roll	Scrambled egg white with Canadian bacon on whole-grain toast
Pork sausage	Turkey sausage, Canadian ham, or center-cut ham
Farina or grits with butter	Oatmeal or hominy grits with margarine
Danish, doughnuts, or croissants	English muffin, whole-grain toast, or low-fat multigrain muffin
Lunch	
Barbecued pork sandwich on white bread or bun	Lean ham or skinless turkey breast on whole-grain bread with mustard
Grilled cheese sandwich with butter	Toasted low-fat cheese sandwich with grated carrots, raisins, or fruit spread for added flavor
French fries	Oven fries, baked potato, or baked chips
Cheeseburger	Plain hamburger with a side salad
Pizza	Vegetable pizza, pizza without meat, or homemade pizza (toasted English muffin with tomato sauce and melted part-skim mozzarella cheese)
Dinner	
Breaded fried chicken or fish	Oven-fried chicken; baked, broiled, or stewed fish
Potato salad	Three-bean salad

Macaroni and cheese	Pasta sprinkled with grated parmesan cheese; homemade macaroni and cheese using low-fat cheese and skim milk
Vegetables prepared with fatback, neck bones, salt pork, or fried vegetables	Vegetables prepared with a small piece of lean ham or smoked turkey; steam vegetables with herbs and lemon
Cornbread	Cornbread made with skim milk and egg white; low-fat bran muffins or whole-grain rolls
Spare ribs	Boneless pork loin or lean stewed beef

Snacks and Desserts

Sweet potato pie	Sweet potato pudding, omit the crust and make traditional whipped sweet potatoes using egg whites, low-fat milk and low-calorie margarine
Rice pudding	Use skim milk and for variety make lemon rice pudding—add grated lemon rind and lemon juice
Ice cream	Sherbet, low-fat frozen yogurt, ice milk, sorbet, or fruit shakes
Frosted cakes or pound cake	Angel food cake with fresh strawberries or gingerbread
Chocolate cookies	Fig cookies, gingersnaps, graham crackers, or vanilla wafers
Candy bars	Hard candy or jelly beans
Buttered popcorn and potato chips	Plain air-popped popcorn, pretzels, baked tortilla chips

and eating to become part of your normal lifestyle. That's how you're going to maintain that lovely weight you've worked so hard to attain.

Of course, even the best of us slip up sometimes. After all, that golden-crisp fried chicken skin is the best part. And you've got to at least taste your niece's wedding cake. But if you slip up, enjoy it. By planning the week's menu this way, you can anticipate some of the situations that may take you outside your own kitchen—and off your *HealthQuest* 30-Day Weight-Loss Program. That way you can plan in advance to get in a little extra exercise or cut a few more calories the day before and after to make up for whatever slip-ups you might have. So if you see that wedding is on the calendar for Saturday, trim a little extra from Friday's menu to give yourself some wiggle room.

Tips for Healthy Grocery Shopping

Here's another reason why it pays to plan your menu in advance: Many people find that, by planning a weekly menu, they can shop more efficiently, buying exactly and only what they need and thus saving money on their grocery bills. But you're gonna have to change your shopping habits. No more standing with your head in the ice cream freezer while your glasses fog up. And we want you to spend less time on the snack-food aisle. Here are some tips to help you shop in a way that will support your lifestyle changes.

• Pick busier stores. They sell more goods, so it's more likely the food will be fresher and more nutritious. That means supermarkets are usually better sources of fresh food than corner stores.

• Shop the perimeter of the store. Fresh produce, meats, and dairy items tend to ring the store. Highly processed foods reside on the inside aisles.

• Use fresh fruits and vegetables instead of canned goods. You'll maximize nutrition while cutting down on sodium. If you can't find fresh food, try frozen instead.

• Pick lean and extra-lean cuts of meat. Select cuts of meat with less visible fat.

• Reduce your reliance on fatback. To season greens and other vegetables, substitute smoked turkey, low-salt chicken stock, or vegetable stock.

• Experiment with turkey sausage and bacon, meatless sausage and bacon, and soy burgers (we love the taste of Boca Burgers).

• Read labels. In chapter 3 we introduced you to the nutrition facts label on most food packaging. Use this information to make informed decisions about calorie, fat, saturated fat, cholesterol, and sodium content of the foods you bring into your home.

Think It Through

You may have thought losing weight was the hard part. If so, you're mistaken. The hardest part of losing weight is keeping the weight off. Remember, 90 percent of people fail to keep the weight off for two years. That's why we suggest you spend six months losing 10 to 15 percent of your weight, followed by some time spent focusing solely upon maintaining the weight you've achieved. This is a time to practice your healthy lifestyle changes so that they become habits. Familiarize yourself with the proper serving sizes of your favorite foods. Practice saving a couple of calories here and a couple there. Shop the perimeter of the supermarket. Negotiate for healthy meals when you eat out. Plan your meals and make shopping lists.

The more you practice these and other healthy behaviors, the more deeply ingrained they'll come and the more likely they'll become healthy habits you'll maintain throughout your lifetime. Once healthy behaviors become enjoyable and habitual, the more you increase the likelihood that you'll be successful if you choose to lose additional weight. In either case, losing weight and keeping it off is cause to celebrate!

For Your Spirit

W hen you first start to make dietary changes, your mind, body, and spirit will go through an adjustment period, especially if the changes are radical. During the first week, you may feel tired and hungry all the time. Your digestive system may feel off-kilter and you may be constipated or have gas. Don't be surprised if you get headaches. Emotionally, you may feel frustrated, irritable, stressed out, and unable to concentrate. If you're the type of person who doesn't have much variety in your diet, you may find yourself feeling bored, deprived, or limited by your food choices. Then again, you may feel tight for time, even overwhelmed, as you're now forced to think about food choices that used to be routine or are trying to incorporate new behaviors into your old way of living. It may become clear to you that it is impossible to make all the necessary changes the way your life is currently set up. Your spirit will be tested. You may feel like something has to give.

All of these feelings are normal. Not only does your body have to adjust to your new diet, it will rush to flush toxins out of your system the moment you stop eating unhealthy foods. That's the reason for some of the unpleasant physical and emotional symptoms; your miraculous body is throwing out the trash and flushing toxins down the drain (don't forget to drink plenty of water). Rather than taking aspirin for headaches or laxatives to relieve the constipation, we suggest you ride out these changes, taking note of them as they occur and observing how they resolve themselves. This is a great chance to get more in touch with your body. The severity of your symptoms merely reflects the degree to which you burdened your body when you were unconscious of the relationship between what you ate and how your body functions. Just try to grin and bear it. Consider the discomfort your body's payback for unknowingly (or knowingly) abusing it.

As you become aware of the level of commitment required to take proper care of yourself, you may start to realize how much our culture discourages a healthy lifestyle—and also how that's starting to change in some places. Notice how the most convenient places to eat often only serve highly processed foods. Try getting a green vegetable in some fast-food restaurants, for instance. It just isn't gonna happen. Observe how the appetizers are prepared at chain sit-down restaurants—most are battered, breaded, and/or fried. On the other hand, many food courts and supermarkets now have a cornucopia of fruits and vegetables available at a salad bar. Some convenience marts carry fruits and vegetables. Bottles of water are now available at most places soda is sold. And some fast-food restaurants even have salad bars and grilled or baked chicken sandwiches.

Make no mistake—the process of changing your diet can require a tremendous amount of work and conscious effort. Depending upon your eating habits beforehand, making these changes may challenge every fiber of your being and put your spirit to the test. You may need to cut back on your commitments and social activities to make time for yourself. You may have to ask your friends, family members, or significant other for help. You'll need to pray for strength, focus, and determination.

But don't despair; your prayers will be answered. You should start to feel better by the beginning of week two, sooner if you're making less-radical lifestyle changes. As toxins get flushed out of your system, you'll transition from feeling hungry and tired to feeling full faster and energized. You'll find yourself urinating more, feeling less bloated, and having more-regular bowel movements. People who have health problems may very well notice their breathing improve, their blood pressure go down, or their diabetes come into control. Your sense of being bored with your food choices may subside, as you step out of your food rut and experiment with new ingredients, recipes (don't forget the ones in appendix 3), and cuisines. You'll start to stumble upon healthy places to eat out and find that some of your friends want to join you.

During the first two weeks that you change your food choices, write about all these changes in your Food and Fitness Diary. Note any discomfort you're feeling, any symptoms of detoxification or other changes you experience. Write and meditate on the miracle of your body. Describe how your body feels as any discomfort starts to subside, how excited and energized you become as these changes build upon themselves and as you start to gain momentum. Now is a good time to congratulate yourself and to thank God that your body is so forgiving and has the power to regenerate itself. You're making it over the hump and are well on your way.

CHAPTER 8

Moving in
a New Direction

Why You Need to Exercise

It's a common scenario: You're following your diet, losing a satisfying pound or two each week. Then suddenly the scale gets stuck. You haven't lost an ounce this week. Next week it's the same. You cut back a few more calories, and wait.

Nothing.

The next thing you do is blame yourself: *Maybe I wasn't doing something right.* Then you get depressed: *I'll never lose all this weight.* Then you're ready to give up and go find yourself a bag of chocolate chip cookies.

Whoa! Back up for a minute. You shouldn't blame yourself. A stalled weight-loss attempt often has to do with your body's physiology. You've got to realize that you're working with a pretty smart machine. It knows it needs food to survive and interprets a reduction in calories as a sign that you might be starving. So when you start cutting back, your body is genetically programmed to slow down your metabolism. That's why you eventually stop losing weight.

Here's how it works: Let's say you're accustomed to eating roughly 2,000 calories a day. Let's also assume that your metabolism burns up 2,000 calories a day. You take in exactly as many calories as you burn, so your weight is stable.

Then one day you take a tip from your homegirl Earline and decide to try the latest fad—Dr. Slim's Stringbean Diet. Now, you like green beans as much as the next person, but you can only manage to throw down 1,500 or so calories worth of the little fellas each day. Still, you're now eating 500 fewer calories than you're burning, and you start to lose weight. After the first week, you've lost nine pounds. "That Dr. Slim's a genius!" you tell Earline.

Before long, though, you notice you're losing less and less weight each week. What started as nine-pound-a-week losses shrinks to four pounds a week, then two. Then you stop losing weight altogether. You're not doing anything differently—you're eating the same amount of string beans every day—but the diet is just not happening for you.

By now your body has slowed your metabolism. It knows it's not getting as much food as it's used to, and so it turns your metabolic flame down low to try to conserve energy. This action reflects the wisdom of human evolution. Thousands of years ago, people whose bodies could slow their metabolisms to compensate for a slim harvest or a poor hunt gained a genetic advantage over those who couldn't—they were literally less likely to starve to death. Your genes still work that way, which explains why folks typically lose weight when they start to diet but find that weight loss usually tapers off and eventually stops altogether.

What's the Point?

Your body resists diets for another reason: your "set point." The fat in your body doesn't flop anywhere it wants to. It's stored in special fat cells that can fill or drain as your body dictates, kind of like your metabolism speeds up or slows down as needed. When you lose weight, fat drains from your fat cells and is burned for energy. No problem so far, right? But this process also triggers the production of an enzyme—lipoprotein lipase—that tells the depleted fat cells to refill with fat as soon as food is available. Some researchers think this finding is pretty good evidence that everyone has a "set point"—a certain weight that our bodies naturally return to even after the most strenuous dieting.

It's a very good thing that these wonderful systems are genetically hard-wired inside of us. They've helped us and our ancestors survive hard times and to return to good health when times get better. But these survival tools also help explain why it can be mighty hard to lose weight by simply eating fewer calories.

Get Smart

How *do* you lose weight, then? By outsmarting your body. Don't look now, but you've got a secret weapon to help you in the battle of the bulge. Researchers say it's the one way—the only way—to circumvent your body's genetic tendency to hold on to every calorie it can get. Your miracle answer isn't exotic, and it's not very expensive. In fact, it's free.

It's *exercise*. Exercise seems to scramble the body's calorie-conservation cues. Even moderate exercise can be enough to override your genes and start depleting your fat cells. When that happens, you lose weight. It's as simple as that.

It's actually even simpler for men. Think about this: Fat tissue burns calories very slowly—slower than molasses in a snowstorm. Muscle tissue, on the other hand, burns them up like nobody's business. Since the average male body contains more muscle and less fat than female bodies do, and muscle is such an efficient calorie-burner, *most men can lose weight simply by eating better*—which means eating fewer calories, especially fewer fat calories.

Women don't have it so easy, though. Which is why, for women who want to lose weight, a good diet and a good exercise regimen go hand in hand. You can't have one without the other. Choosing broiled fish instead of chicken-fried steak for dinner but skipping your after-dinner walk is better than eating poorly and *not* exercising—but it won't help you drop pounds steadily. On the other hand, working yourself into a sweaty tizzy on the dance floor, then stopping by JB's Soul Shack on the way home is better than not exercising and eating poorly, but it won't do much to wither your waist. For women at least, eating well *and* exercising is the key to successful weight loss—and successful weight management. (Of course, brothers should be exercising, too, to stay healthy and fit.)

What's a Person to Do?

Just like there are two parts to losing weight—dieting and exercise—there are multiple aspects to exercise—stretching, aerobic exercise, and strength training. And you'll do all three as part of your *HealthQuest* 30-Day Weight-Loss Program.

While it may not seem particularly exciting, *stretching* is fantastic exercise. It keeps your body limber and protects against some of the symptoms of aging. And it's especially good for those of us who are older, very overweight, have never worked out before, or have allowed ourselves to get out of shape. But while stretching helps condition your body, it doesn't burn an ounce of fat. You need to do something that works your heart.

Aerobic exercise is where the action is. It's the NBA playoffs we watch on TV, the track meets your kids participate in, the rhythmic movement we see scantily clad models perform as they entice us to join the latest gym. Sports and other energetic activities are aerobic in nature, but the definition of aerobics is very broad; it includes anything that works your heart and lungs. That's why it's often called cardiovascular exercise—"cardio" for short. But while aerobic exercise burns fat, it doesn't sculpt, strengthen, or tone your muscles. That's where the third component of fitness comes in.

Strength training—also called weight training or weight lifting—builds, lifts, and shapes your muscles. It also offsets some important effects of aging, like the loss of strength, bone density (osteoporosis), balance, and coordination. When you see male models with perky pectorals or video queens with tightly sculpted thighs, you can bet that they've been pumping iron. Weight training has even become popular in senior citizen circles because developing strong muscles helps to keep your bones strong and prevents osteoporosis.

Can you see where this is headed—and why it's important for you to participate in all three? Stretching makes your body flexible, aerobics starts the calories burning, and strength training helps you build your muscles. Then the more muscle tissue you build, the faster you burn calories—and the faster you burn calories, the faster you lose weight. That's why the most successful weight-loss programs for women incorporate all three aspects of physical fitness.

Exercise has other important benefits, as well. It conditions your heart, reduces your LDL ("bad") cholesterol level, prevents some types of cancer, boosts your immune system, and lifts your mood. It's like a wonder drug that makes you healthier physically and mentally—with no nasty side effects.

Since exercise is so essential to shaping a new you, we're going to teach you about all three components of exercise and help you develop an exercise regimen to accompany your dietary changes. Until then, start looking for easy and enjoyable ways to add more physical activity to your life. Walk whenever you can, take the stairs, or turn on your favorite song and start dancing. Exercising can be a lot of fun when you have the right outlook about it.

It's All in Your Head

By now you've probably heard that the brain is the most powerful sex organ. It's true: The physical reality can be influenced by your mind's ability to create and transform, imagine, and innovate. If it's not happening in your head, it won't happen in your bed.

The same is true when it comes to exercise. If you have a background in athletics, enjoy sports, or simply love moving your body, then you probably already know that fitness and exercise aren't just a physical thing. Top performers in virtually any sport will tell you how important mental preparation is to successfully working with your body. For example, competitive athletes of all stripes visualize reaching the end of a race or the concluding minutes of a game; they know that "pre-seeing" success helps to guarantee it in real life.

That's true of any activity or goal—perhaps especially losing weight. You need to see it—if only in your own mind—to believe it. (Which is why we asked you earlier to do the exercises visualizing yourself at your ideal weight.) The same is true of exercise.

If you're overweight, however, you may find that imagining *winning* a race isn't really the issue. It may be difficult to envision exercising at all, much less enjoying it enough to do it again, not to mention crossing somebody's finish line. It can be challenging to begin to reconceptualize yourself as a person who *moves*—especially if you're too big to move comfortably, if you feel awkward about even being seen in exercise clothing, if you've never really seen yourself as an active or particularly athletic person—and especially if you've been discouraged from exercising because of your size. It can be challenging to lay aside that hurt and conditioning to begin to see yourself as someone who works their body—who walks or lifts weights or does aerobics or swims and gets sweaty and feels sore and loves their body right along with everyone else.

Trust us, though. When you learn to think of yourself as an exerciser (or as an athlete, even!), you'll be amazed at the transformation that will come over you. Over time, simply thinking of yourself differently can slowly transform any reluctance you may feel to exercise. And once you're exercising, visualization can help keep you motivated from the first minute of your workout to the last.

Nice try, you're saying. *But I'm a couch potato from way back. I never liked exercise when I* had *to exercise*. Maybe you grew up in a house where no one did any physical activity, or where everyone was exercising—except you. Maybe you were the last to be picked for the kickball team. Perhaps the thought of that blue gym suit makes you shudder.

There are a lot of circumstances that could turn you against exercise. We also understand that "exercise" as we think of it now is not naturally a part of everyone's life. Until recently, most folks worked at physically demanding jobs. Black folks, especially, worked hard at backbreaking labor from chopping cotton to hefting heavy washtubs to double-shifting in factories. We also walked to work (or at least to the corner to catch the bus), washed our clothing by hand (or at least lugged them to the laundromat), chopped wood for the fire, and got up off of the couch to change the television channel. Nobody talked about working out; we were too busy *working*.

Back then, we got exercise as part of our day-to-day lives. But these days many of us drive to work, sit behind a desk all day, have lunch delivered, come home and microwave our dinner, then reach for the remote control. We barely have to lift a finger.

So, if you're not all that interested in athletics and you're not naturally getting any exercise in your daily activities, it may be difficult to think about how you might develop good fitness habits at this late date.

Yet there are hundreds of forms of exercise—from bowling and basketball to synchronized swimming and spelunking (that's cave exploring). There's golf, dancing, skating, karate, tennis, archery, skiing, gymnastics, boxing, diving—you name it. Surely there's some form of exercise that you'd like to learn and would enjoy doing. And maybe it's not feasible to go scuba diving three times a week, but we're going to help you find something that's convenient, enjoyable, and appropriate for your budget and your temperament.

Think It Through

When it comes to moving the body, you've got to move the mind first. The following questions will help you explore your feelings about exercise and begin to liberate the active, athletic person who lives within you.

Childhood Memories

Close your eyes for a moment and think back to some of your earliest memories of exercising your body. You might remember yourself riding a bike, playing baseball, rolling down a hill, jumping rope, or doing sit-ups in gym class. Then, in each category below, select the sentence that best describes you and write it in your Food and Fitness Diary.

- I liked to play outdoors.
- I preferred inside games and activities.

- I enjoyed playing with other people.
- I had fun with solo activities.

- I felt at ease playing and exercising.
- I felt awkward when I was doing something physical.

- I was always snapped right up when people were choosing teams.
- I hated/dreaded team selections; I was always the last to be chosen.

- Someone/everyone in my family was pretty fit and active.
- I grew up with a low-key bunch; we didn't do much physical activity.

- My favorite playtime activities were (list physical activities as well as other types of games):

Current Reality

Looking back at our childhood interests can remind us of forgotten dreams and the simple pleasures that brought us joy. Sometimes these memories give us a peek inside the window of our heart's desires. But regardless of your history, part of getting involved in an effective exercise program is learning what turns you on today. Yes, you do have to get moving, but you don't have to do anything you don't want to do. Answering the following questions will help you figure out what kinds of exercise options you might enjoy.

- I'm pretty competitive and I'm motivated by winning.
- I like to do things where I can challenge myself.

- I like to do things that allow me to feel graceful.
- I like things that make me feel strong.

- I would like to have some muscle definition you could see.
- I want to be fit, but I don't have to be chiseled.

- I want to see results fast.
- I can afford to take my time to reach a good fitness level.

- I'm self-motivated. Once I set my mind to it, no one can stop me.
- I like working with someone so we can support and motivate each other.

- How much can you spend on fitness?
  - Nothing. It's not in my budget.

- Under $100 one time for some at-home equipment.
- $30–$50 a month to join a gym or take weekly classes.
- Several hundred for home gym equipment or a personal trainer.

Once you've completed the questions in both sections, take a look at your answers. When you look at them all together, you'll begin to see some patterns and preferences emerge. Record your thoughts in your fitness journal. They will be instrumental in helping you identify the right fitness program for you as we begin to examine the different types of exercise in the following chapters.

For Your Spirit

We're going to practice visualization again—this time to help us imagine what it feels like to be comfortable in physically active bodies.

Find a quiet and comfortable space, and call on your imagination. Close your eyes and visualize your body in motion. What would you be doing if you were a comfortable weight and you enjoyed being active in your body?

Picture yourself as active as you ideally want to be. Would you be indoors taking an exercise class or outdoors frolicking in the warm sun? Is there a childhood desire you're still longing to fulfill—to be a ballerina or play on the basketball team? Or maybe you'd like to make fitness a family affair and sign up for karate classes with your kids or take walks together after dinner. Have you always wanted to explore the great outdoors—perhaps by going canoeing or riding a mountain bike? Maybe you've envisioned yourself on a tropical island, skimming across the waves on a windsurfer, hiking along a volcanic trail, or performing yoga on the sand at sunset.

Let your mind run wild and free. Let your imagination clear the couch potato cobwebs and bring in crisp and refreshing change. Make sure to write down your thoughts in your fitness journal. We'll come back and use them later.

CHAPTER 9

STRETCHING THE LIMITS

A Full-Body Stretching Routine

If you don't know much about stretching, you're in very good company. It's the Rodney Dangerfield of physical fitness, the component of exercise that just gets no respect. The popular perception in the United States is that while stretching is probably beneficial, when it comes to real fitness, it's nothing to get bent out of shape about. But in other parts of the world, people widely understand that yoga, tai-chi, and other stretching exercises contribute significantly to their overall health and wellness.

In spite of our cultural preference for more exciting forms of exercise, stretching ranks right up there with aerobic exercise and proper nutrition as a factor in sustaining wellness and achieving a fitness lifestyle. The American College of Sports Medicine, the definitive source on fitness matters, recommends that we integrate stretching into our lives no less than three days a week.

Since stretching is such a fantastic form of exercise and an easy place to start if you're older, overweight, or have been inactive, we've made sure to include it in the *HealthQuest* 30-Day Weight-Loss Program. In this chapter, we will provide you with a full-body stretching routine. We'll also introduce you to yoga, one of the most popular forms of stretching, as well as to tai-chi and to Pilates. Use stretches as a gentle way to get to know your body and ease it into motion in a way that isn't embarrassing or painful—no matter your size or fitness level. This routine can be done in the privacy of your home and you don't need to own anything made of spandex.

What's So Good About Stretching?

The benefits of stretching may surprise you. For starters, it's a great way to get in tune with what's going on inside your body. If you have never exercised before, stretching will give you a better feeling for how your foot bone's connected to your anklebone and your anklebone's connected to the shinbone. In the process of feeling these connections, you'll also become aware of the places in your body that are holding tension. That's important for all of us to know, because internalized stress can set the stage for disease. If you've never worked out before or if you have gotten out of shape, you'll also begin to feel the light aching and tingling sensations that accompany the process of lengthening your muscles and causing the blood to circulate within them.

In addition to helping you get in touch with your body, stretching protects against some of the symptoms of aging. Our tendons, which connect our muscles to our bones, begin to shorten as we grow older. As a result, our joints lose their full range of motion, move less easily, and we become less flexible. You may have watched this happen to an older loved one or even felt it in your own body—maybe you're starting to feel stiff in the mornings, have difficulty touching your toes, or are not as limber as you used to be. Over time, this loss of flexibility can cause us to look and feel older than our age, as we develop poor posture and lose our ability to stand up straight or to extend our legs to full stride.

Another benefit of having a flexible body is that you're much less likely to be injured while exercising, if you lose your balance or experience a bout of clumsiness. But perhaps the best thing about stretching is that it's an equal-opportunity activity. You can stretch no matter your age, weight, or fitness level. It's cost-free, fun, and can be done anywhere, whether you're working out, at your desk, behind the counter, on the assembly line, or stuck in a marathon meeting.

How to Stretch

Most people incorporate stretching into their fitness routine in one of two ways: They stretch as an exercise regimen in and of itself, or include it as part of their aerobic or strength-training workout. Either way, you should stretch for ten minutes a day at least three times a week, and preferably five times. If you follow this suggestion, stretching can slow, even prevent, the process of aging by restoring the range of motion your body used to have.

But as gentle as the motions are, before you start stretching you have to warm up your body. You wouldn't start driving your car without first starting the engine and letting it warm up for a while and you shouldn't do so with your body, either. Just like your car, your body needs a moment to warm up before you begin to exercise.

Warming-up literally increases your body temperature. Warmer muscles, joints, and tendons are more limber and pliable and, therefore, less likely to strain or tear. (That is why it's so important to warm up before you stretch.) The warm-up also signals to your body that it's time for it to redirect the flow of blood to the large muscles that will help you move your body. This is especially important when you're just starting out, because your body isn't accustomed to supporting those muscles and can get confused about where it's supposed to send the blood. If you experience a passing sensation of light-headedness, that's probably what's happening; you don't want to find out the hard way by falling out. So take five to fifteen minutes to warm yourself up; brisk walking, riding a stationary bike, or using a climber or stepper, such as the StairMaster, are all good options. You'll know that your body's warm when you break into a light sweat. At that point you can safely proceed with your aerobic workout.

When you finish your workout you should do a *cooldown*. The cooldown is just the opposite of warming up. It tells your body to redirect your blood back to your stomach, colon, and the other places it normally goes when your body isn't being exerted. The cooldown also prevents your blood from pooling in your legs or other parts of your body, leaving you feeling light-headed and faint at the end of your workout. If you weight-train or engage in a cardiovascular workout, you should stretch between exercises and also when you finish, while your muscles are still warm, limber, and pliable.

Before we introduce you to the workout itself, let's spend a moment reviewing some stretching technique. First, know that the act of stretching should consist of slow and gentle movements. This is contrary to what many people have been taught. Many of us have learned to bounce as we stretch, but this is a time when having "more bounce to the ounce" can cause muscle tears or pulls.

Many of us have also learned to stretch to the beat of the music. Music can inspire and motivate us, but if we focus on it instead of what's happening in our bodies, we lose some of the benefit of the exercise. Stretching is a mind-body exercise, an opportunity to connect our minds to what we feel inside our bodies. Use this time to get in tune with yourself. For instance, as you're stretching, notice whether your muscles and joints feel soft, limber, and pliable; tight, resistant, and uncooperative; or someplace in between. Do you feel them lengthening and supporting you, or are they signifying and asking if you've gone out of your mind? If you feel tightness, is it symmetrical or only on one side? Is it in the muscle or in a joint? Can you identify what that tightness might be from— holding the telephone with your shoulder, too many hours on your feet? These are the types of things to become aware of when you engage in a stretching routine.

When you stretch, hold each position for from twenty to sixty seconds. Relax as much as you can and breathe deeply, pulling fresh air into the bottom of your lungs. Then envision directing your breath into any places that feel tense or tight. For instance, if your hamstrings are tight, imagine your lungs extending into the back of your legs. Then imagine your muscles loosening and softening. The more frequently you stretch, the more you will begin to feel any resistance subside and you will be able to relax farther into each stretch. But stretch only as far as feels comfortable, and remember: Don't bounce, whatever you do.

After your workout don't be surprised if your muscles give you some lip and talk back to you by feeling sore, achy, or tender. Soreness is your body's natural response when you work your muscles in new and different ways. It will probably peak within two days and slowly subside from there. Just reach into the back of the closet, pull out the Epsom salts, and draw yourself a warm bath like Granddaddy did. Or maybe it's time to treat yourself to some fragrant bath salts; you probably need an excuse to pamper yourself, anyway.

Your spirit may give your some lip, too—especially if you're not used to flexing your spiritual muscles in this area of your life. For instance, spiritual resistance may come in the form of not feeling motivated to continue your stretches. This is the time to pray for strength and determination or to repeat your affirmations (for instance, *I am enjoying the process of becoming more healthy*). Another great way to motivate yourself is to meditate on the ancestors. Imagine how sore our ancestors must have felt as they performed the backbreaking work of picking cotton, for instance. Their ability to activate their spirits to overcome spiritual, mental, and physical pain and degradation is what allows you to be reading this book in comfort today. Ask our Creator to imbue you with the fighting spirit our ancestors had. You'll get over your hurdles in no time.

Full-Body Stretch Routine

Here's a basic stretching routine covering all the major muscles, giving you a dynamic full-body stretch, from your calves to your neck. Don't be surprised if you feel awkward at first or if your body feels uncooperative. That feeling will go away as your body gets used to the movements. Before you begin each stretch, read the instructions carefully and look at the positions in the photos.

Neck Stretch

This stretch has three movements and should be done while sitting in a chair. Sit erect with your chest forward; your shoulders should be back and relaxed. Place your feet flat on the floor.

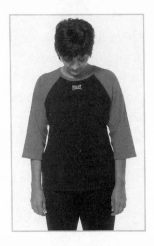

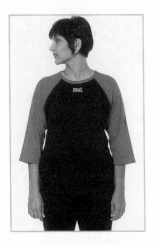

Slowly lower your chin toward your chest. Hold until you feel the stretch. Gently return your head to the starting position.

Keeping your chin up, turn your head completely to the right without moving your shoulders. Hold and feel the stretch. Return to the neutral position, head upright and facing forward.

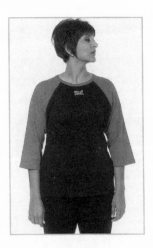

Then repeat on the left side.

Shoulder Stretch

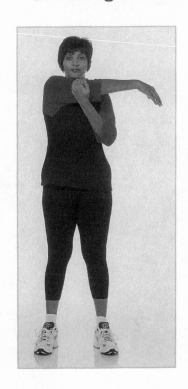

Stand up straight with your feet shoulder-width apart. Pull your right arm across your chest about chin high. Hold your head in a neutral position. Place your left hand on your right elbow and press slightly. Hold. You should feel tension in your right shoulder. Repeat on opposite side.

Tricep Stretch

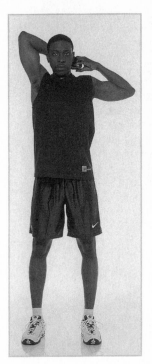
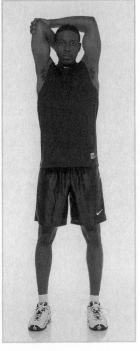

Stand up straight with your feet shoulder-width apart. Place your right hand behind your head on your left shoulder. Grasp your right hand with your left hand. Use your left hand to pull your right elbow toward your head. Hold. You should feel tension behind your upper right arm. Repeat on the opposite side.

Upper Back and Chest Stretch

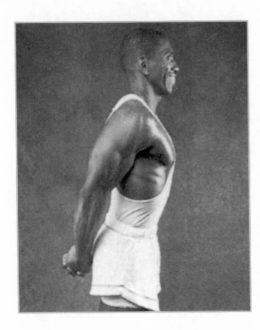

Stand up straight with your feet shoulder-width apart. Keep your head in a neutral position and clasp your hands behind your back at waist level. Keep your chest up and shoulders back. Slowly lift your arms behind you until you feel a squeeze in the middle of your back. Hold. Slowly release. This stretch is also good to release slumping shoulders.

Quadricep (Front of Thigh) Stretch

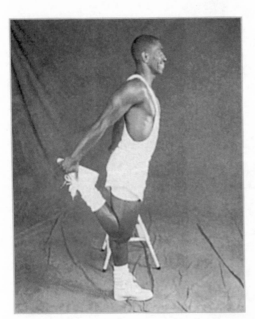

Stand up straight next to the wall, a chair, or other sturdy object to support yourself. Put your feet close together. With your right hand, reach back and pick up your right ankle. Bend your left knee slightly and drop your right hip. Now slowly pull right ankle up toward your behind. Hold. Switch legs and repeat.

Hamstring (Back of Thigh) Stretch

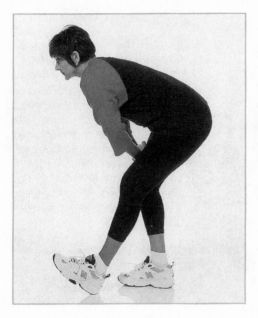

Stand with your feet shoulder-width apart. Place your right leg straight in front of you with your heel on the floor and toes pointed upward. Bend forward, keeping your back straight. Place your hands on your thigh just above your left knee. Now bend at the left knee until you feel the stretch in your right hamstring. Switch legs and repeat.

Calf Stretch

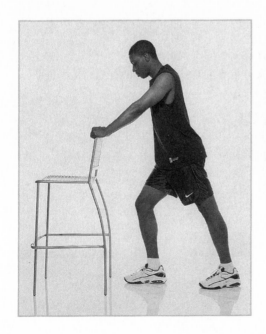

Using a wall, chair, or something sturdy for support, stand with feet shoulder-width apart and pointed straight ahead. Place your left foot behind you but keep your heel flat on the floor. Now bend your right knee and move your hips forward, like you're about to push a car. You should feel tension in your left calf. Keep your head facing forward. Hold. Repeat using your right foot.

Lower Back

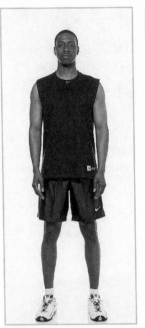 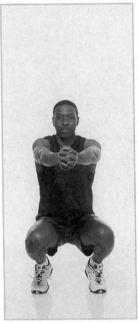

Stand erect with your feet shoulder-width apart. Keep your head in a neutral position and extend your arms shoulder high. Now clasp your hands in front of you with your palms together. While reaching out in front of you, slowly bend at the knees. Bend until your thighs are parallel to the floor. Hold. Release your arms and slowly return to upright position.

 Stretching Dos and Don'ts

Stretching looks easy, but if you want to reap the full benefit, you've got to do it right. Follow these tips to get the most out of your stretching workout.

DO:
- Stretch three to five times per week and after every cardiovascular and strength-training workout.
- Pay attention to how much tension you feel, as well as any soreness in your muscles.
- Hold each position for twenty to sixty seconds and feel your muscles stretching.

- Breathe slowly and deliberately throughout the stretch. Feel your chest cavity swell, then gradually let the air out.
- Stay focused and in tune with your body during each movement.

DON'T:

- Overdo it; move slowly and gently. If a precondition or past injury causes discomfort, pain, or aggravation, don't stretch at all.
- Stretch muscles when they are still cold. Warm up first with five minutes of nonstop movements (try marching in place, jogging, vigorous housework) until you break a light sweat. Warm muscles are more pliable and easier to stretch.
- Bounce, jerk, or rush to achieve a deeper stretch. These movements can injure tendons, ligaments, joints, and muscles.
- Stretch too far. Stop before it feels uncomfortable.

The Home Stretch

If you like stretching, you may also enjoy these other popular mind-body techniques that can be done at home or at a gym.

Pilates

Pronounced *pih-LAH-teez*, this is a conditioning program performed on mats or special Pilates machines that stretches and conditions the core of your body: your lower back, abs, buttocks, and thighs. The exercises focus on developing your strength and teaching proper body mechanics, so it will help you develop good posture, as well. It's offered in special Pilates studios (www.pilates.com), yoga studios, or in large gyms—but take a mat class for about ten dollars per hour; at sixty dollars per hour and up, machine classes and private lessons can be very expensive. Another option is to rent or buy a videos on Pilates.

Tai-Chi

Pronounced *ty-chee*, this is an ancient Chinese exercise, stress management, and body-awareness technique consisting of slow, gentle, and flow-ing movements, performed with precision and emphasizing proper technique instead of power. Tai-chi is so slow and gentle that it looks like it's being performed in slow motion, but it's really teaching balance, concentration, strength, good posture, flexibility, and body control. Because it's so gentle, it's especially good for seniors. Tai-chi is offered at larger health clubs and martial arts and yoga studios.

Yoga

A series of strength, flexibility, and body-awareness poses intended to strengthen the relationship between mind, body, and spirit. For more on yoga, see "For Your Spirit" at the end of this chapter.

Think It Through

This exercise is designed to help you identify obstacles that could prevent you from embarking on a fitness program or to keep you from being active as often as you should. Think about any resistance you feel to exercising or things that may stand in your way. If any of the following problems ring a bell, the suggested solutions may help. If you have other concerns, write down your obstacles and spend a few moments thinking of a way to head them off before they gain a lot of momentum.

1. *I'm not motivated.*

   - Choose a fitness goal that's especially important to you and imagine how good it will feel to approach it.
   - Set fitness milestones and reward yourself when you reach them.
   - Reread chapter 8!

2. *I'm embarrassed by my size.*

   - Remember that exercising is a form of self-love. You're not doing it for other people. You're doing it for you.
   - Keep in mind that you have a right to be healthy regardless of your weight.

- Remember: It's infinitely preferable to be large and fit than to be thin and out of shape. Everyone has to do the right thing by their body; you're doing what you need to do for yours, and that's all that's important.

3. *I'm new at this. I'll feel awkward.*

- Remind yourself that all new skills are learned gradually. Just like you learned how to ride a bicycle or to use a word processor, you'll get better at exercise the more you practice it.
- In your fitness diary, keep track of how awkward each day's workout feels. See if you gain confidence over time. Our worst fears often dissipate once we confront them and face them openly and honestly.

4. *I have asthma (heart condition, etc.) that requires me to be careful when I exercise.*

- Talk to your doctor about how best to incorporate exercise into your lifestyle. Usually she'll want you to exercise and can help you find a form of physical activity that's healthy for you.
- Realize that your diet may help ease your other symptoms. For example, some experts say that reducing or cutting dairy from your diet can help ease asthma symptoms. Since it also cuts the fat from your diet, you get two benefits for the price of one.

5. *I was hurt once and have ongoing joint problems. I can't move that well and I'm afraid it will flare up again.*

- Physical activity, done safely, can actually help ease joint problems like arthritis. Swimming, low-impact aerobics classes, and other forms of exercise can pamper your joints.
- You can—and should—start out slowly. But the more you move, the better you'll be able to move.

6. *I want to exercise, but I never seem to have time.*

- Get up a fifteen minutes earlier in the morning and do some jumping jacks, a few sit-ups, some squats, or other exercises. Exercise doesn't have to be a big production.
- Take a walk on your lunch hour. Thirty minutes is plenty of time to eat; use the rest of the time for a brisk stroll.
- Use your exercise time as additional time to spend with your kids. Take them on a powerwalk through the park, or play a rousing game of tag in the yard. Many gyms offer a babysitting service; look into this option.

List as many other obstacles as you can think and brainstorm of ways to talk yourself through them. Remember, the key is to be affirmative.

For Your Spirit

Stretching Your Limits

If you're receptive to an unconventional fitness approach that's steeped in spirituality, consider yoga, a practice that seems to appeal to more and more African-Americans every year.

The word "yoga" means "union"—as in the union of the mind, body, and spirit—and there are several different forms of the practice. Many African-Americans are introduced to the practice through Hatha ("sun and moon") yoga, which emphasizes bringing your entire system into balance through right action, thinking, breathing, eating, meditation, and devotion. And within Hatha yoga, there are several varying techniques.

Yoga is based in the theory that by practicing certain breathing techniques and doing special body postures, you can rejuvenate and revitalize the body and cultivate a wonderful sense of mental and spiritual well-being. Hatha yoga postures, called *asanas*, provide specific ways of stretching that elongate and strengthen your muscles and massage your internal organs, from head to toe. Yoga's deep-breathing techniques increase the supply of oxygen to the body. Working together, they increase relaxation and improve circulation, digestion, respiration, and elimination. They also rejuvenate your internal organs and strengthen the immune system.

In those senses, yoga resembles aerobic exercise. But yoga differs from typical workouts. For example, in many forms of exercise, you're trying to reach a goal—a certain amount of laps swum, miles biked, weight lifted. They are future goals—and they can bring a degree of the tension that comes when we're trying to achieve something. In yoga, you learn to relax into the posture, just doing whatever your body allows in the moment. In this noncompetitive mind-set, you can relax mentally as well, and healing can occur.

Yoga is a fascinating blend of contrasts. It can be aerobic; it can be still. It can be uncomfortable; it can be comforting. It can be demanding; it can be gentle. But it always serves to make you more aware: aware of your body, aware of your hidden emotions, aware of what you eat, aware of how you're sitting or standing, aware of your breath, aware of your patterns of thinking, and, most important, aware of your right on this earth to be healthy and happy.

You can take yoga classes at many gyms and YMCAs, through continuing education programs, or at studios especially for yoga. If you're not ready to make that investment, pick up one of many good yoga books, magazines, and videos on the market. Find one that offers instruction for beginners and try a few of the asanas and breathing exercises. A few tips:

• *Don't be intimidated by pictures of models that look as if they're molded from rubber.* They've probably been doing it for years. You can get benefits from yoga without being a contortionist.

• *Don't feel bad if you can't quite touch your toes yet.* It takes time to ease your body into doing new things. Yoga is an exercise in patience and encourages you to be patient with yourself.

• *Don't think that you have to be as thin as a yogi to do yoga.* You'll be surprised at how limber you can become once you start moving your muscles. Even before you reach your desired weight.

Here's an example of a yoga exercise that's good for relieving neck and shoulder tension, a major cause of headache:

1. Sit comfortably at the front edge of a chair with your feet flat on the floor, arms hanging at your sides. Sit tall yet relaxed, letting all of the tension out of your shoulders. Hold your head in a neutral upright position. Softly close your eyes as you begin to breathe deeply. Relax your body from feet to head, silently naming each body part as you exhale and relax it. This should take about thirty seconds. Take five deep breaths in this relaxed state.

2. On your next exhalation, let your chin fall to your chest. Continue to breathe deeply. Relax all the muscles in your face and begin to slowly swing your chin from side to side, feeling the sensations in the back of your neck. (To take this movement a little deeper, interlace your fingers and place your hands on the back of your head, bringing your elbows toward each other. Do not pull your head down; just allow the weight of your hands and gravity to bring the head closer to the chest.) Remember to breathe deeply. To release the posture, first return your hands to your lap, then slowly bring your head back up to a neutral position. Stop and notice how you are feeling before you begin the next movement.

3. Next, begin a counter-movement by gently and slowly allowing your head to fall backward. Allow your mouth to open and make sure your shoulders are relaxed. Take five deep breaths in this position. As your eyes remain closed, gently lift your head back to the center.

4. To continue to relax and stretch the muscles in your neck, just allow your right ear to fall toward your right shoulder, noticing and exploring the stretch in the left side of the neck. To deepen this stretch, allow the right arm to come up and cradle the head as your right hand gently lays on top of your left ear. Hold this posture for ten to fifteen seconds, breathing as you go. To release, drop the arm back down to your lap, gently inhale, and raise your head back to center. Repeat on the opposite side. Remember that the key to releasing tension is to inhale deeply and exhale fully.

CHAPTER 10

Work That Body!

Understanding Aerobic Training

By now you've probably started to incorporate stretching into your lifestyle and are becoming more aware of how flexible you are (or aren't). You're certainly not the Rubber Band Man—at least not yet!—and it's possible that you haven't even completed the full-body stretching routine. But perhaps you're stretching a bit when you get up each morning and a couple of times during your day at work. You're becoming more aware of the places in your body where you hold tension. And you're feeling those delicious aches and pains that come from bringing rusty and underutilized body parts alive. So now you're ready to move to the next step—the part where you burn calories by exercising and you really start to lose weight. That's where aerobic exercise comes in.

In this chapter, you'll learn about aerobic exercise and the role it can play in burning fat. We'll introduce you to a number of aerobic workouts and give you the pros and cons of each of them, so you can decide which are right for you. You'll also start to create some exercise goals.

But don't start panicking! If you're one of the many people who doesn't particularly care for aerobic exercise, we'll help you build up to it one step at a time, starting with a hip new exercise called walking. We'll tell you about a good friend of ours, Connie, who lost 109 pounds and went from fat to fit when she started walking and became encouraged about eating right. If she can do it, you can, too.

What's Aerobic Exercise?

As you learned in chapter 8, aerobic exercise includes any repetitive activity that gets your heart pumping and lungs breathing deeply.

For this to happen, you have to repeatedly work the large muscles of your body, including your behind, thighs, legs, and chest.

What kind of exercise is aerobic in nature? Well, clicking the computer mouse with your right forefinger is certainly a repetitive movement, but it doesn't work your major muscles, so surfing the Internet doesn't count. And though you do work your butt and thigh muscles when you bend over to get the skillet so you can fry up a pork chop, we certainly hope it's not a repetitive motion. What does count is anything from walking the treadmill to using a LifeCycle to taking Tae Bo to playing football to modern dancing to chopping down a tree to shoveling snow. You can see that there are a wide variety of ways for you to get aerobic exercise throughout the day.

Our objective is to get you involved in an aerobic activity for at least thirty minutes a day, at least five days a week (you should always take a day off). But you'll lose weight faster if you work out aerobically for at least forty-five minutes. This is because the human body doesn't start to burn fat until about the twenty-minute mark. The good news is that you don't have to work out for forty-five minutes straight; several ten-minute bursts throughout the day will yield the same results. But you do have to exercise consistently. Remember: you're trying to burn at least 250 calories. The more you burn, the faster you'll lose weight. And the more intense your workout, the quicker you'll burn calories.

How do you know how hard to work out? The "talk test" is a great way to measure how hard you're working. While you're exercising, you should be able to engage in a conversation without feeling as though your lungs are going to burst like a birthday balloon. You're probably not working hard enough if you can sing all the words to Michael Jackson's "Thriller" in the middle of your spinning class (although you're probably in good shape if you're able to do all the moves). But if you can't catch your breath long enough to tell your workout partner to slow down, you're probably working a bit too hard.

So now that you understand the basic principles behind aerobic workouts, let's take a look at the various types, starting with walking, a great place to begin the exercise component of your *HealthQuest* 30-Day Weight-Loss Program. We recommend walking for everyone, particularly if you're older, severely overweight, or out of shape.

One Step at a Time

Connie B. (not her real name) weighed 279 pounds the morning she decided that enough was enough. She donated her bathroom scale to charity. "Hey, I figured I'd give it to the Salvation Army, because it sure wasn't 'saving' me."

She had been trying to lose weight for years, especially after the birth of her son left her with twenty-five extra pounds that went right to her middle and stayed there. As her weight grew steadily each year, she became more depressed, which led her straight to her favorite snack: pound cake and coffee. Some days she would put away two Sarah Lee pound cakes, she says—and be looking around for more. "I just couldn't get enough of it," Connie remembers. "It was a terribly lonely and desperate time for me."

Not that Connie didn't try to fight back. She tried every new diet she heard about. She lost eight pounds on the Lemonade Diet, but she could only manage to stay on that for three days before surrendering to her cravings for real food. She gave the Cabbage Soup Diet and the Grapefruit Diet a spin—and they worked for a while. Eventually, though, she grew so sick of eating one food that she abandoned her restrictive eating plans to save her sanity. And as soon as she went back to her old eating habits, she gave it up. Sometimes she even regained a little more than she had lost. Talk about doubly depressing.

Connie had never been all that fond of exercising. Anyway, she says, she didn't have many role models. "I used to tell my girlfriend Marlene—she weighed about the same that I did at the time—that all I saw out there doing aerobics was skinny girls who look like they don't even need to exercise," she recalls. "Do you see anyone in those skimpy little outfits who looks like us?"

But one day in August, Marlene phoned Connie excitedly to tell her of a new exercise program the church was starting. A few women had formed a walking club and they were looking for others. When Connie heard that the women were beating the summer heat by walking in a nearby mall, it was hard to say no. She could check out the fall fashions and do something good for her body in one fell swoop. So she and Marlene laced up their sneakers and joined their friends.

Today, Connie calls it the best decision she's ever made. The women walked every afternoon for thirty minutes after work, and they made small but significant changes to trim the fat from their diets, eat fewer empty calories, and eat more vegetables, beans, and fruits. She held on to her beloved pound cake, but she switched to a low-fat version and decided to try and enjoy normal serving sizes.

In the first few weeks at the mall, Connie felt awkward about her size. And it wasn't easy to move a reluctant body that had grown accustomed to staying put. But she stuck with it. By August of the following year, she had lost sixty-five pounds—and kept it off. Connie was pleasantly stunned by how wonderful she looked. "Brothers started to turn their heads when I walked past, and friends would pass me on the street and not recognize me," she recalls. Most of all, she says she's grateful for how good she feels. Her anguish over her size has been replaced with a new sense of confidence and calm, and the various aches and distresses that were an everyday part of living in her old body have vanished into thin air. Now that she's lost 109 pounds and reached her target weight of 170, Connie still eats well and walks daily. It's her ticket to a better life, she says, and she's not about to give it up.

Getting on the Good Foot

Like Connie, thousands of Black folks nationwide are discovering that good health can be as easy as putting one foot in front of the other. Since 1990, walking has been the first choice of fitness enthusiasts, according to a survey conducted annually by the National Sporting Goods Association. More than 60 million folks have made it their exercise of choice. So let's examine the benefits of walking before we check out the other varieties of exercise available to us. Why are so many people so hyped about walking?

First of all, anyone can do it. You don't need to be twig thin or able to contort your body into the shape of a pretzel. There's no jumping and hopping around; you don't have to be coordinated, have rhythm, or learn steps; and you don't have to worry about getting hurt.

Going the Distance

How do you know how far you're walking? Depending on where you decide to walk, there are a number of ways to calculate the distance. If you plan to walk in a park and are willing to follow an exercise trail, the distance may already be measured for you. Look for distance markers along the side of the path or a map of the park that shows the distance between milestones. If you'd rather walk in a neighborhood, first identify the route you'd like to walk, then drive it in your car, measuring the distance on your odometer. In many areas, especially cities, the length of each block is about the same; eight blocks to the mile, for instance. (Don't forget to measure the short side of the block in addition to the long side.) You can measure the distance in your car or, if you take the bus, ask your favorite driver to help you.

Walking can also improve your health. It relieves stress and increases your sense of well-being, helps prevent osteoporosis, and makes your bowel movements more regular. It can also combat life-threatening diseases like heart attack and stroke by helping reduce cholesterol and blood pressure levels.

It's a good way to create a healthy support system. Just ask Hughrine West, who talked to *HealthQuest* magazine about her participation in a Walking for Wellness group in Baltimore. The women in her group discuss their children, careers, dilemmas, and triumphs. There's also a chance to network, she says. And within the group women find support for the healthy lifestyle choices they've made.

Walking is easy on your wallet. "All you need is a good pair of walking shoes—and motivation," says Charles F. Reid Jr., a personal trainer in Clarksdale, Mississippi. Many people walk in sneakers, although you may want to invest in walking shoes that cushion your feet, legs, and hips against hard asphalt and concrete (and get padded socks if you really want to pamper your feet). A decent pair of walking shoes will run you $60 or less. Compare that to the prices of gym memberships, bicycles, step machines, treadmills, or even skates.

It's easy on your nerves. One of the benefits of walking is getting outside and breathing a little fresh air. But not all of us live in a neighbor-hood that feels safe, and women walking alone need to be especially care-ful no matter where they walk. So if you don't feel comfortable walking outdoors, try an indoor mall, track, or treadmill, where you can walk to your heart's content year-round in warmth and perfect safety. Many malls open their doors early—even before the stores open—so that early risers can get their walk in.

It's tough on fat. Just because walking is easy on the body doesn't mean it's soft on fat. A leisurely stroll at three miles per hour burns about 290 calories per hour—about the same as pulling a golf cart or taking a slow bike ride. Walking more briskly at four miles per hour burns around 400 calories an hour. That's equivalent to roller skating or cycling at ten miles per hour. And when you up the pace to five miles per hour, you burn 460 calories an hour—the same level of exercise as water skiing or singles tennis. Any way you slice it, walking can really put a hurting on a bunch of calories.

But while walking is an affordable, efficient, low-impact exercise with high-impact benefits, it's not everyone's cup of tea. When you're looking for a way to lose weight and boost your health, you need to find some-thing you like. And even if you enjoy walking, you may want to mix it up a bit. "When people think that exercise is a chore, they won't stick with it," advises weight trainer Reid. "If you don't enjoy walking, find some-thing else to do."

 You'll Never Walk Alone

Theresa Kello of Boston was on the brink of developing hypertension when she and about twenty of her coworkers started a chapter of Walking for Wellness, a program created by the National Black Women's Health Project. As a result of her walking effort, Kello's blood pressure eventually normalized. Georgia M. Sharpe, co-leader of the walking club with Kello, says that walking helped improve her diabetes. She needed less insulin thanks to her walking regimen.

How can you hook up with a group so you can enjoy walking's benefits? These resources can help you get started.

The American Heart Association's Choose to Move is designed to help women become more active. Call 1-888-MY-HEART for more information.

The National Institute of Diabetes and Digestive and Kidney Diseases (NIDDK) has established the Weight-Control Information Network (WIN) to assemble and distribute information on weight control, obesity, and nutritional disorders. WIN has published *Sisters Together: Move More, Eat Better* a planning guide to help organizations create programs to help Black women control their weight. The good news is, it really works. The program is based on a three-year health-awareness program held in Boston. Call (877) 946-4627 or (202) 828-1028 for more information.

Your church. Many churches are implementing fitness programs. Check with the head of your health or fitness ministry to get their help in starting a walking group. The Heart Association or WIN information can help you get going.

A World of Options

So what else *is* there to do? You name it. Aerobic exercise covers a huge territory, from rowing to in-line skating, badminton to basketball, swimming to skating. If you're an indoor exerciser, there's stair-climbing, stationary bicycling, and working the treadmill. If you're sweet on the great outdoors, there's hiking, canoeing, kayaking, and cross-country skiing. If you play racket sports well enough to work your body continuously, there's tennis, racketball, and handball. Remember: Any exercise that's rhythmic and continuous, and that involves your large muscles and that gets your heart pumping steadily for at least twenty minutes counts as aerobic.

All you have to do is figure out which exercise is best for you. Below you'll find a chart to help you weigh the pros and cons of a number of popular exercise routines. Each type of exercise is accompanied by an estimate of the number of calories that a 150-pound person will burn in an hour. The best aerobics workout consists of activities that become a regular part of your life because you enjoy doing them. It will challenge you mentally and physically, but feels like a challenge you can meet

Exercise	Pros	Cons	Calories/hour
			150 lb. person
Aerobics (Hi/Low Impact, Funk/Hip-Hop, Step)	Good cardiovascular workout; strengthens and tones muscles	High-impact classes can be hard on joints. Look for low-impact and step classes.	475
Baseball/Softball	Fun way to get active if anyone's any good.	You end up standing around a lot, particularly with beginners. There are much better workouts.	340
Basketball	Great cardio workout for people who are already in shape.	Hard on aging muscles and joints, especially knees and ankles. If you're not in shape, shoot baskets, but don't compete.	545
Biking (road and mountain)	Good cardio workout; strengthens legs, especially quadraceps.	You need a bike, a helmet, and a safe place to ride. Because the bike, not your bones, supports your body weight, it doesn't protect against osteoporosis.	375, leisurely; 475, moderate or stationary bike; 680 fast pace
Boxing Aerobics/ Tae Bo	Excellent cardio workout, tones and strengthens muscles.	Take an instructional class first, so you don't injure yourself.	660
DANCING			
African	Good cardio workout; works entire body.	Warm up thoroughly; intricate moves.	305, but depends on type of dance and intensity of effort
Ballet	Increases agility and flexibility.	Can cause joint injuries. Best to be in shape.	
Hip-Hop	Increases strength, posture, and balance. All ages.	Can feel rigid and overly structured.	
Jazz/Modern	Excellent aerobic workout; stomach, behind, thighs.		
Salsa	Good cardio workout; increases strength and flexibility, especially in legs and torso. Tightens tummies, thighs, and tushes.		

Gardening	A great way to commune with nature.	Watch out for those thorns!	340
Golfing	Gets you in touch with nature. Exercises mental discipline. Walking the course is good low-impact exercise.	Walk the course, don't take the cart. And watch out for incoming balls. Fore!	375, assuming you walk and carry your bag
Karate/Martial Arts	Promotes mind/body awareness; strength; self-discipline.	Getting whupped by little kids can be hard on your pride.	368
Mowing the lawn (power walk mower)	The smell of fresh cut grass.	The smell of fresh cut grass.	305
Pilates	Strengthens back and abs; improves posture and flexibility; mind/body connection.	Take a mat class; individual sessions are expensive.	272
Racquetball/Squash (casual)	Great cardio workout; improves hand-eye coordination.	Be careful of joint injuries.	475
Raking leaves	A clean lawn. Good upper body workout.	Depends on how many trees you have.	270
Rowing	Great cardio workout; strengthens the total body.	Requires a boat and a river unless you do it at the gym.	415
Running	Great cardio workout; burns lots of calories; strengthens lower body; you can do it anywhere.	Can be hard on knees, shins, and ankles. Many people develop chronic injuries.	680 at 6 mph (the same as a 10-minute mile)
Shoveling dirt	A great upper body workout that builds physical and cardio strength.	Watch your back!	580
Skating (Ice, In-Line, Roller)	Builds balance and lower-body strength, especially thighs.	Requires skates, plus a helmet and pads. Falls can be wicked.	475
Soccer/Football (casual)	Excellent cardio workout; strengthens lower body.	Requires a field and a team.	475
Spinning	Excellent aerobic workout; strengthens lower body.	For some people the seat can be uncomfortable until you get used to it. Ouch!	680

Exercise	Pros	Cons	Calories/hour
Stair Climbing	Great cardio workout and calorie burner; strengthens butt and thighs.	Can become monotonous, so mix it up. Some people experience knee problems.	610
Swimming	Excellent aerobic workout; strengthens and tones the entire body. Great for people who are injured, pregnant, arthritic, or obese. You may even save a life.	Oh, go ahead and get your hair wet! If you're modest, a nice towel or wrap will cover you until you get into the water. If you can't swim, use a kickboard. Doesn't protect against osteoporosis because your body weight is supported by the water.	545
Tai-Chi	Excellent mind/body workout; promotes inner peace; great for seniors, those new to exercise, and anyone who doesn't want to sweat out her curls.	If you like action, tai-chi will be a snoozer.	272
Tennis	Great cardio workout; strengthens and tones entire body.	Watch out for injuries to your wrists, knees, ankles, and shoulders.	475
Walking/Hiking	Strengthens and tones lower body; easy to sustain; low injury rate.	Some people find it boring. If the weather's bad, your streets are busy, or the neighborhood isn't safe, go to a park or the mall.	292, assuming 15-minute mile on a flat surface
Weight Lifting	Strengthens entire body; helps prevent bone loss.	You can purchase a number of weights for under $50.	205
Yoga	Excellent mind/body workout; strengthens and tones entire body; promotes sense of overall peace.	Be patient, you don't turn into a pretzel overnight.	170

because it is geared to your level of fitness, your age, and your interests. It's rewarding because it's safe, effective, and achieves your physiological, psychological, and spiritual goals.

Aerobics or Aerobics?

The term "aerobics" refers to a component of fitness, but it's also used to describe a very popular type of exercise class. Aerobics classes are offered at every school, gym, and community center, and are a great way for a beginner to get physically fit. If you've ever taken aerobics before, you already know what to expect. But if you haven't, deciding which class to take can be a bit intimidating.

Aerobics classes are choreographed exercise classes led by a certified instructor that are designed to work your heart, lungs, and major muscle groups (therefore, the term "aerobics"). They usually consist of a warm-up, the exercises themselves, a cooldown and stretching. Many classes also include an abdominal workout, so be prepared to bust a gut! They're also a great place to make friends, learn basic body mechanics, how to use hand weights, and take your pulse properly.

We recommend that you observe several classes first. But even then, you are likely to leave with a misimpression; it will look to you like everyone knows all the moves, but many of the participants have been taking aerobics for years. So make sure you talk to the instructor, too. Let them know if you've ever worked out before and what fitness goals you have for yourself. They can help you decide if theirs is the right class for you and will help you get started during the first couple of classes. But even before you venture out to the gym, you'll want to know a bit about the different aerobics classes.

High-impact classes are often moderately paced, but usually involve hopping and jumping around (think "jumping jacks"). The classes are great if you're coordinated and already in shape, but can be challenging if you've never done them before. In *low-impact* classes, you'll always have one foot on the floor. That makes it easier for heavier folks and those who are less coordinated or are new to working out. *Funk* or *hip-hop* classes draw on music video style dance moves, but depending upon the class, may require that you're in video shape. If you can find a beginner's class or if you can hang with the hip-hop homies, you'll learn you have muscles you never knew you had. *Step* aerobics involves doing choreographed moves on and off of a rectangular plastic step (the gym will provide it). You determine the height of the step, from about four inches up to about a foot. In addition to working your heart and lungs, these classes also tighten your tush.

At the Starting Gate

So you're pumped, right? You're motivated, you're educated, and you're ready to hit the gym (or sidewalk, or pool, or . . .). Before you head out there and make your mark, here are a few tips to help you develop a safe, effective, and most of all *enjoyable* aerobic exercise program. Bear these in mind when you start the aerobic exercise component of your *HealthQuest* 30-Day Weight-Loss Program.

• *Begin at the beginning.* Before you begin a fitness program, consult your doctor, consult your doctor, consult your doctor. We can't say it enough—especially if you are extremely overweight or have any sort of chronic health condition. So mark this section in the book and take it with you to your doctor's appointment. Make sure to talk to the person who provides you with health care, who knows your health history, and can give you sound advice. Ask them to help you figure out how much exercise is appropriate and what types of exercise might be right for you.

• *Do what you like.* There's not much point in torturing yourself with an exercise that you really don't care for, so find an exercise that you enjoy and go to town with it. You can even get some of the benefits of strenuous exercise from gardening, if you can believe it. Bottom line: Whatever you like to do, go ahead and do it.

• *Set aside enough time.* You lead a busy life, we know. But try not to rush through a workout. Savor it as *your* time, a special time of the day when you can be good *to* yourself and do something good *for* yourself. Count on devoting at least an hour for your workouts—less when you're just starting out. And remember: several smaller aerobic workouts—five to fifteen minutes long or fifteen to thirty minutes long—within a twenty-four-hour period are just as effective as one continuous thirty- to sixty-minute workout.

- *Exercise frequently.* Exercise benefits your body the most when you do it routinely, not sporadically. If you've been sedentary for a while, go easy on yourself and start slowly with five- or ten-minute workouts, but do them consistently five or six times a week. Studies show that's the ideal frequency for losing weight. You'll eventually be able to add more time to the workout until you're doing thirty minutes or more per day.

- *Be consistent.* To be effective, your workout doesn't have to leave you gasping for the paramedics. But it must be consistent—occasional or sporadic workouts won't do much to help you lose weight or condition your heart. (You can see the value of choosing an activity that you like, right?) If you're a reasonably disciplined person, you won't have much trouble setting a fitness schedule and sticking with it. If not, go ahead and set a workout plan in motion, anyway. In fact, you may enjoy it so much that you decide to make aerobic exercise a part of your regular routine.

- *Set some fitness goals.* Decide where you want to be, fitness-wise. We'll talk about this more at the end of this chapter.

- *Start s-l-o-w-l-y.* Don't forget your five- to ten-minute warm-up. Whatever your exercise, do it slowly and at a low intensity for a minute or two. If you are walking, for example, gradually walk a little faster, lengthen your stride, and swing your arms more vigorously until you reach your target heart rate. You'll know that your body is warm when you break into a light sweat.

- *Monitor the intensity of your workout.* If you work out at a gym, you'll notice people watching a clock while touching a pulse point. That's how athletes monitor how hard their heart is working. But your *HealthQuest* 30-Day Weight-Loss Program frees you from a number of conventional exercise chores, and this is one of them. Don't worry about your pulse rate. Instead, take the "talk test." Remember: If you're breathing hard but you can carry on a regular conversation, you're exercising in the moderate range. If you're breathing so hard that you can't converse, you've crossed over to the intense range. You can keep moving, but don't overdo it.

• *Cool down.* End your workout with a five- to ten-minute cooldown. Use the same slow, low-intensity movements that you warmed up with.

• *Stretch.* Stretch, slowly and deliberately, after the cooldown phase of your exercise program when your muscles are most limber and less prone to injury. Pay special attention to the muscles you used in your workout. For example, if you were walking, be sure to stretch your calves, thighs, hamstrings, and heel cords. Hold each stretch for twenty to sixty seconds, then relax. Breathe slowly and deliberately; avoid holding your breath. Plan to stretch for five to fifteen minutes, depending on your fitness level. If you're a novice, go for the full fifteen minutes.

• *No shortcuts.* Don't count your warm-up and cooldown minutes as part of your aerobic exercise. For example, if you walked for a total of forty-five minutes, including a five-minute warm-up and a five-minute cooldown, your total aerobic workout time was thirty-five minutes.

• *Mix it up.* Alternating between high-, low-, and nonimpact activities lessens your chance of injury. For example, you might walk or do low-impact aerobics on Monday, Wednesday, and Friday, and cycle or swim on Tuesday and Thursday. This is called aerobic cross-training. Cross-training reduces the risk of overusing your muscles and joints, decreases the possibility of boredom, and adds variety and challenge to your workouts.

• *Be patient.* Research suggests that a slow, consistent, well-paced progression toward your fitness goals is the best way to obtain and maintain long-term health changes.

Think It Through

Creating Exercise Goals

If you're like most people, you'll probably find that exercise gets easier the more you do it. It's like moving a train out of the station: It's hard to get the thing rolling, but once it goes, it has momentum of its own. Many people find that exercise becomes nearly effortless as their body gets better conditioned and increasingly used to the new demands that exercise places on it, and as exercise becomes more and more a part of their everyday routine, just like brushing their teeth in the morning. In tandem with good eating, once-hesitant pounds just begin to melt away.

But if you haven't been working out, you're going to need to take it slow. Research shows that if you've been sedentary, it can be dangerous to jump into a vigorous workout program right away. So don't let your good intentions backfire on you. You probably need to start out by cutting more calories from your diet, rather than burning a whole lot of calories with exercise.

Then again, don't start to think that because of your heart condition or your arthritis or your age, you're going to be given a reprieve from exercise. Everyone can do *something*. And no matter what your health condition is, exercise—in some form or the other—is likely to help it. It's just a matter of approaching your fitness program appropriately: with patience and common sense. So we're going to start setting some exercise goals.

Scoring Goals

What are your fitness goals? It may not sound like an important question, but unless you establish a goal, how will you know why you're working out? How will you know when you've finished one phase of your work and it's time to move on to the next phase? And on those chilly winter days when it's hard to get out of bed, much less get to the gym, how will you remind yourself of the reason you're doing all of this in the first place?

Different exercisers are driven by different motives. Your primary goal is probably to lose weight. But here are some additional very common—and very achievable—fitness goals that work hand in hand with weight loss. Do any of these apply to you?

I want to work out:

- to feel less stressed out.
- to feel better about myself.
- to give me more endurance.
- to bring down my blood pressure.
- to increase my HDL cholesterol (the good stuff).
- to decrease my LDL cholesterol (the bad stuff).
- to bring more calm into my life.
- to heighten my sense of spirituality.
- to improve my circulation.
- to help me use less insulin (for diabetics).
- to lift my mood.
- to have some quiet time to myself.
- to help me be less anxious.
- to provide a social outlet.
- to just feel healthier and more fit.
- to feel more confident
- Others:

Next, you're going to create some goals. You'll make your goals as *specific* as possible. Be descriptive and use numbers, dates, times, and other *measurable* characteristics. That way you'll have something to shoot for and feel good knowing that you achieved it. In appendix 4 we'll give you planners so you can record your progress.

It's important to make sure that your goals are *achievable*. You won't feel good about yourself if you set yourself up to fail. If you haven't exercised in the past six years, it is not reasonable or healthy to expect to run a half-marathon in two months. You also want your objectives to reflect the other priorities in your life. If you're starting to exercise at the same time you're starting a new job, chances are that exercise scheduled for after work during the week will lose out. You might want to work out in the mornings before work or schedule extra time to exercise on the weekend in case you miss a workout during the week.

Ask your doctor to help you create exercise goals that reflect the state of your health. Or try some of these goals on for size:

To exercise for thirty minutes a day for five days a week (three times during the week and twice on weekends).

To be able to do the StairMaster for forty-five minutes straight by my birthday four months from now.

To be so flexible that I can bend over and touch my toes by the thirtieth of this month.

To jog one mile within two months.

For Your Spirit

Zoning Out

You may have heard athletes talk about being "in the zone." When basketball players are in the zone, they say they can pass and shoot the ball effortlessly, moving with assurance and grace on the basketball court without having to think about it. Tennis players talk of tuning out the noises of the crowd and other distractions, and seeing nothing but that fuzzy yellow ball. Walkers, cyclists, and runners get so into the flow of motion that they sometimes lose track of what their legs are doing!

Being in the zone is wonderfully pleasant and satisfying. Your spirit soars, you lose track of time, and you forget whatever worries may have been pressing on you just a few minutes before.

Exercise physiologists say there are upwards of one hundred physical benefits of exercise—benefits like having a more efficient cardiovascular system, a heightened immune response, and stronger bones. But the spiritual benefits of exercise are formidable, too. When you've exercised long enough to get into that zone, you feel relaxed, content, and at peace with the world. It's the state that many athletes—professional and amateur alike—treasure the most about their workouts. And who wouldn't want to feel that good?

So, how do you get to be in the zone? It's not hard. In fact, it begins to happen naturally after twenty to thirty minutes of continuous rhythmic exercise. When you get moving, the brain produces endorphins—natural opiates produced in response to exercise and other stresses. Those endorphins are feel-good substances that have a lot to do with lifting exercisers into the zone.

Continuous exercise means you keep moving for a specified time without stopping. So tennis isn't continuous the way most of us play it; unless you're pretty good at it you probably spend as much time hitting the ball as you do walking over to the fence to pick up balls you've missed. If you're a good biker on an uninterrupted path, that's continuous. "Rhythmic" means you're moving with a steady beat—like jogging, swimming laps, dancing, stair-climbing, and step aerobics, among others. As you begin to add regular exercise to your daily schedule, notice the many spiritual benefits you enjoy.

You will feel more alive as you breathe deeply and blood courses through your veins, supplying nutrients and oxygen to your pumping muscles. The soreness in your calves, that stitch in your side, and the callus on the ball of your foot are signs that you are alive and that your body is taking steps to support the newly active you.

You will notice that any depression, numbness, or lifelessness you may be experiencing within your life will slowly begin to lift. You will start to experience a sense of overall well-being.

If you exercise outdoors, you will find yourself becoming more in tune with nature—the sounds of birds chirping, the bright glint of sunlight off a freshly fallen snow, the earthy aroma of autumn leaves.

You will notice sluggish thinking disappear, that your head feels clear and your worries dissipate. Your ability to focus at work will improve.

The more you incorporate exercise into your schedule, the longer you'll find its benefits will last.

CHAPTER 11

Staying Strong

Weight Training to Tone, Sculpt, and Burn Off the Pounds

As you've been learning and, hopefully, experiencing, exercise can be fun as well as rewarding. We assume that you've started, even perhaps in just taking baby steps. Your muscles may be a little sore and achy. But if you've been working out, stretching is already making your body more flexible, aerobic exercise is accelerating your fat-burning metabolism, and your spirit is certainly becoming stronger as you motivate yourself to overcome obstacles. However, neither stretching nor aerobic exercises tone your muscles very effectively. That means that your body isn't burning fat as fast as it can. For that, you need something that will work with aerobics to send pounds packing. It's called strength training.

Many of us aren't very familiar with strength training. And even if you do know a little bit about it, weight lifting may not seem like something you can relate to. Instead, you may think about "dumb jocks," steroids, and bodybuilding competitions—but that's not all there is to it.

In strength training, you challenge your muscles with physical resistance, using your own body weight, free weights, weight machines, or elastic resistance bands. The resistance challenges your muscles, thereby strengthening and toning them. Toned muscles speed up your metabolism, sending your calorie-burning ability into overdrive.

In this chapter, we'll teach you about the difference between free weights and weight machines, and tell you what you need to know to set up a home gym. If you belong to a health club, we'll decode the cryptic language of the weight room, so you'll feel more comfortable venturing in there. And we've also included instructions for sixteen strength-training exercises for the gym or at home that will help you tighten your tush, sculpt your stomach, and beautify your biceps, all while burning away our nemesis—fat.

In the next chapter, we'll give you two workout routines for your use. One routine is a full-body workout that needs no special equipment and costs nothing. This routine is made up of exercises that work your entire body and utilize only your body weight. The other routine is designed to be used with weights—barbells and dumbbells—and can be done at home or in a gym.

You've Got the Power

You may think that strength training is the last thing an overweight person needs to do. After all, strength training *builds* your muscles and everyone knows muscle weighs more than fat. If you're a man, you may aspire to look like you're in the World Wrestling Federation, but what woman wants to make her body more bulky? Well, lifting weights does add strength to your muscles and may even add a little bulk, but it also increases the amount of muscle tissue, which burns calories more efficiently than fat.

Strength training works by speeding up your *metabolism*, the number of calories your body burns when you're resting and it's performing basic functions, like operating your organs, regenerating new cells, and making your hair grow. The rate of your metabolism is determined by the amount of your body that's free of fat, including muscles, organs, bones, and skin. Since you can't make your brain any bigger or become any more big-boned than you're already claiming, and since nobody wants extra skin sagging down, the only remaining option is to increase your muscle mass. (Remember: Muscles are why men lose weight more easily than women.) For every pound of body weight that you convert from fat to muscle, you increase your metabolism by 10 to 15 calories per day. Now, that may not seem like much, but saving calories is a lot like clipping coupons or pinching pennies; they can really add up.

Say you convert five pounds of body fat to muscle instead. Your body will burn an additional 50 to 75 calories per day. That's a *minimum* of 18,250 calories per year, the equivalent of about six pounds that your body will burn off or you won't gain. On the upside, you could burn about nine pounds. Every year. All from lifting weights. This doesn't include the weight you lose from aerobic exercise or changing your diet! By increasing the proportion of muscle tissue to fat tissue, you gradually convert your body into a lean, mean, calorie-burning machine. It also gives you a little wiggle room if you want an occasional slice of pecan pie.

Aside from losing weight and the obvious vanity benefits—think sculpted shoulders and six-pack abs—strength training is great for other reasons. Like aerobic exercise, it helps strengthen your heart, lungs, and circulatory system. Lifting weights also strengthens your bones. (The more you can lift, the more you stress your bones, and it is exactly this stress that stimulates them to become stronger.) When your body is strong, you become more sure-footed and less prone to injury. And although they're a long shot for most of us, did we already mention the marvel of six-pack abs?

Building Your Strength

There are three parts to a strength-training workout: exercises that focus your upper-body muscles—working your chest, back, shoulders, and arms (biceps, and triceps); those that focus your lower body—working your legs (quadriceps, hamstrings, and calves), hips, and buttocks; and those that work the midsection (upper and lower abdominals and your obliques). We'll incorporate all three into our weight-training program. (And remember: Your weight-training program is meant to be *in addition* to your aerobics and stretching routines. We'll show you how to incorporate all three components to your weekly workouts in the next chapter.) If you are older or very overweight, or have not exercised in a long time (or ever before), you should do, at the very minimum, at least one exercise for each body section twice a week. Everyone should work up to weight training for at least twenty minutes, two to four times a week, preferably doing two or more exercises for each body part.

Four days a week! Won't that make me muscle-bound or keep me from fitting into my clothes? Not likely. Think about Janet Jackson's transition from chunky to svelte and tightly toned; she's much smaller than she was before. And she achieved this by incorporating a weight-training program into her regimen.

Still, if you work any given set of muscles hard enough, yes, you can overdevelop them. That's not our objective, though. Our goal is to implement a balanced weight-training routine that works a number of muscle groups rather than building one muscle to the exclusion of others. When you exercise your muscles this way, you won't start to look like a bodybuilder, although you will certainly look more sculpted and less round.

Along the way, you'll progress through several stages. The first couple of times out, you may struggle to get through the routine or to control the weight. Afterward your muscles will probably feel very sore (remember that box of Epsom salts?). Don't worry; the soreness will diminish as your muscles get stronger and more skilled at exercise and lifting weights. During this time you'll also notice your body becoming more powerful. This may happen gradually or you may become significantly stronger from session to session. At about the eight-week mark, the size of your muscles will begin to increase. Even then, they'll get larger slowly and are much more likely to become shapely, instead. By the end of ten to twelve weeks, you may be 10 to 40 percent stronger than when you started.

Talking the Talk

L ifting weights is a lot like going to school; once you master certain information you pass to the next grade—only in strength training you're graduating your muscles instead of your brain. Just like school, it has its own vocabulary. And it relies on the concept of repetition. In fact, the main idea behind strength training is to repeat the motion of lifting a weight until you exhaust the muscle you're working. Over time, that muscle will get stronger. When the exercise no longer challenges and tires the muscle, you increase the amount of weight and continue doing the exercise at the higher weight level.

Since each exercise requires that you repeat a lifting motion, it makes sense that each time you lift a weight it is called a *repetition* or *rep*. For each strength-training exercise you do, plan on lifting the weight for eight to fifteen reps.

Each group of reps is called a *set*. You should do between two and four sets of every exercise. So say you're doing the exercise called the "chest press." Your first set might consist of twelve to fifteen reps, then you'll do another set of twelve reps, resting for no more than two minutes between each set. When you complete your second set, you can move on to the next exercise.

Most people strength train using either *weight machines* or *free weights*. If you train at home with weights, you'll rely upon free weights, unless you want to invest in some pricey equipment. (We'll assume you'd rather lift weights on the cheap.) If you belong to a gym, you can do either or both. Weight machines and free weights both work fine and you do basically the same exercises whichever approach you choose.

Weight machines are precisely that, machines with handles that are connected to chains or cables, which in turn are connected to weights. When you push or pull on the handle of the machine, the weights (called *weight plates, plates, weight stacks,* or *stacks*) move up or down. You change the amount of resistance your muscles encounter by increasing or lowering the amount of weight.

There are many advantages to using weight machines. They place your body in the proper position and restrict your range of motion, so machines are easier for beginners to use and reduce the likelihood they'll hurt themselves. The machines are often arranged in the gym in the order in which you should do the exercises (this sequence is called a *circuit*), so you can usually move through your regimen quickly (circuits can take as little as twenty minutes). But weight machines have seats, settings, and other things that need adjusting. That's one of many reasons you should have a trainer help you get started (you should also enlist the help of a trainer the first couple of times you lift free weights). Weight machines are very predictable, so they can get a little boring. And you're not going to be able to do them at home, so you may want to learn to lift free weights as well.

The phrase *free weight* refers to barbells and dumbbells, not to their price, although they're often inexpensive. The "free" means the weight isn't connected to a machine. *Dumbbells* are short bars with weights on either end. A dumbbell is designed to be held in your hand. *Barbells* have a long bar between the weight plates at either end. They're used to lift heavier weights (the bar itself may weigh thirty-five pounds or more) so must be held with both hands. You can change the weight by sliding plates on and off the end of the bar.

There are a number of advantages to training with free weights. Free weights are more versatile than weight machines. You can use the same eight-pound dumbbell to do a variety of exercises, whereas each weight machine can only work one part of your body. Because there's no machine to guide and control your motion, when you lift and lower the weight, you expend extra effort to keep it steady. So each lift of a free weight uses more muscles than the exact same exercise on a weight machine. As a result, most people find that free weights make them stronger faster than weight machines and do a better job of sculpting their muscles. You can buy dumbbells weighing as little as two pounds, and they're very inexpensive. The downside to free weights is that they're a little bit harder for a beginner to learn, since there's no machine to guide your form and movement. As a result, you need to make sure to use proper form; otherwise, you can injure yourself. (So pay close attention to the weightlifting instructions later in the chapter or have a trainer help you get started.)

Weight Room Rules

If you want to lift free weights and belong to a gym, we can't emphasize enough the importance of asking a trainer to help you get started. Not only are free weights more difficult to use than weight machines, when you don't know what you're doing, it can be very intimidating to be in a room full of people working so hard that they're grunting and snorting. Your trainer can also help you learn the ropes.

Now, there's a certain protocol people follow in a weight room, but no one will tell you about it until you mess up. In that respect, going to the weight room is a little bit like going to church. At church, everyone knows when to sit, sing, stand, and recite, and there are certain rules that you should follow if you get there late. But if you've never been to church before, you may barge into the sanctuary in the middle of a prayer—and you know what type of looks that's likely to bring, even in the house of the Lord on Sunday!

Just like at church, most people in a weight room are very friendly and there's a camaraderie that develops between the regulars. People may be very focused in the weight room because they're working hard. So don't annoy them by asking an endless number of questions or trying to engage in a lot of chitchat. "Working out" is just that—*work*. And most people need to stay focused when they work. Having said that, it is okay to ask for help when you need it—and at one time or another, you certainly will.

Once you're standing in the weight room, you'll notice that most of the dumbbells and weight plates are housed on racks. Always return them to the racks after you're finished. If you see dumbbells sitting out on the floor, chances are that someone is using them and has put them down while they rest, so ask before you walk off with them. If you want to use the same weights someone else is using, ask if you can "rotate in" with them. That means you'll lift while they're resting and they'll work while you're resting. Don't take it personally if someone says no; it probably means they're very focused or are working with a partner.

And by all means, if you're having trouble lifting a weight, be certain to ask someone for help. Weight lifters will gladly help you get a plate on or off a bar. And if your exercise calls for lifting a heavy weight, feel free to ask someone for a "spot." That means they'll stand next to you to give you assistance if the weight gets too heavy and you're having trouble lifting or putting it down safely. The last thing you want to do is get hurt. (And ALWAYS exercise caution when lifting heavy weights at home alone.)

Creating a Power House

To weight train at home with free weights, you'll need to make a modest investment in some equipment. That will allow you to do most of the same exercises you can do at the gym.

First, you'll need to purchase several pairs of dumbbells. Depending upon your fitness level, you may want to start with weights as low as two to five pounds, but it won't take long until you're using eight- to twelve-pound weights. Eventually a woman will be able to lift fifteen to twenty pounds in each hand and a man will be able to lift twenty-five to forty pounds. Not to worry, though, you should be able to purchase eight sets of dumbbells for somewhere between fifty and one hundred fifty dollars. And if push comes to shove, you can use a bottle full of water (1.5 liters equals three pounds) or take that same container and fill it with sand. If you do this, be very careful when you lift, since these containers weren't designed with weight lifting in mind. And be particularly careful not to strain your wrists.

You'll also need a flat weight bench, preferably one that also inclines and has thick foam padding on it. They are available at sporting goods stores for one hundred to three hundred dollars. If you don't have that kind of money, you can do several of these exercises using a chair, piano bench, or picnic bench. It helps to have access to a set of stairs. And you'll certainly want a full-length mirror to make certain you're using the proper form—and to admire your body once you begin to make progress!

How to Get Started

Whether you strength train with machines or free weights, at the gym or in your home, follow these guidelines for getting started:

• Beginners should complete one to two sets of eight to fifteen reps for each strength-training exercise they do. If you're more advanced, work up to three to four sets of fifteen reps each, then move up to a higher weight.

• Try to find the balance between too much weight and too little. You do this by fine-tuning the amount of weight with the number of reps; the weight should be heavy enough that the last repetition is a struggle—but not so much of a struggle that you lose your good form or technique. For instance, if you can chest press eight pounds twenty times, that weight is too light. Move up to ten pounds and see if you can lift it fifteen times, keeping good form. If so, increase the weight to twelve-pound dumbbells. If not, keep lifting the ten-pound weight until, over time, you can lift it fifteen times without breaking your form. Then move up to the twelve-pound dumbbells.

• Count to two as you lift each weight and count to four as you lower it. Don't let the weights bang when you get to the top of your motion. And don't stop to rest at either the top or bottom of your motion.

• Rest for about a minute and a half in between sets.

• It doesn't matter what muscle group you start out with—your chest, back, or legs. But work your larger muscles before you work the smaller ones. For instance, work your back muscles, chest, and thighs before you do your biceps, triceps, or calves.

 You Want Results?

Two words: *Pushups* and *Squats*. If you do nothing else, be sure you do some pushups and some squats. These are the two single most effective strength-training exercises you can do for working your upper and lower body respectively, along with some benefit to your midsection.

Pushups work every muscle group in your upper body and require abdominal control, working your midsection as well. You'll feel these in your chest, back, shoulders, and arms. Not to worry if you can't do a traditional off-the-floor pushup, because we'll tell you how to start doing these from off a wall, until you get stronger and stronger, progressing lower and lower to the floor, until you're capable of doing a full pushup routine. (See the "Perfect Pushup" box on page 193.)

Squats work all the muscle groups in your lower body and, like pushups, also require abdominal control for your midsection. You'll be working your butt, hips, thighs, and calves, and using all the multiple joints of your lower body (your ankles, knees, and hips). (Squats are explained in the section on lower-body exercises, on page 200.)

These two exercises will work all the major muscles groups in your body, at the same time strengthening your minor muscle groups as well, so they're not only effective, they're time-efficient.

Strength-Training Exercises

Now that you know the basics of strength training, it's time to give lifting weights a try. Remember: You want to do at least one exercise from each category at least two times per week. Ideally, you'll choose at least two exercises from each category and lift more than twice a week.

Upper-Body Exercises

Flat-Bench Dumbbell Flys

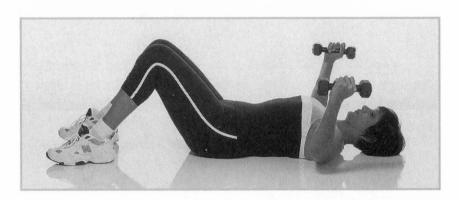

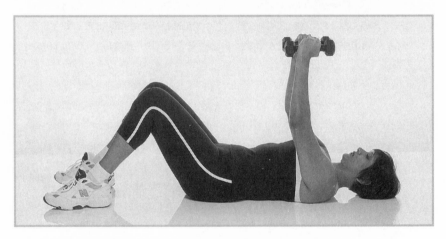

Primary muscle group worked: Pectorals (chest).

Lie on your back with your knees bent, feet flat, and lower back flat against the floor or on a bench. Hold your dumbbells above your chest with your arms extended and elbows slightly bent. Your palms should be facing each other. Lower the dumbbells in a semicircle away from the center of your body. Keep your elbows relaxed and away from your torso. Exhale and bring the weights back to the top of the circle. Note: As you raise the dumbbells, make a conscious effort to flex your chest. The movement spreads your chest when you lower the weights. It takes inner-chest strength to pull the weight upward.

The Perfect Pushup

Pushups primarily work the pectorals, or chest muscles. But they also strengthen shoulders and work your arms, particularly your triceps if you do them using a narrow grip or with hands close together. The tightening of your midsection when you control the pushup also works your abdominals and helps to firm this area as well. If you can't do the Traditional, Basic Pushup, start out by doing the Wall Pushoffs described below. Then progress to an Incline Pushup (stabilizing yourself from a low bookcase, sofa, or chair), then on to the Modified Pushup, where you'll do your pushups kneeling. Using this method, you will eventually work your way down to the floor and will be strong enough to begin a routine of Traditional Pushups, when you'll attempt to do more pushups faster. This is truly the best exercise that you can do to build upper-body strength.

The Traditional, Basic Pushup

Lie face down on the floor with hands slightly wider than shoulder width apart and palms flat on the floor. Legs should be straight and toes tucked under the body. Straighten your arms as you push your body off the floor. Exhale as you push and keep head and neck in one line and your body parallel to the floor. Then bend your arms and lower your body until your chest almost touches the floor, keeping your back straight.

Do as many as you can until you reach failure or you lose your form. If you reach failure before completing three sets of fifteen repetitions, finish your pushup routine using Modified Pushups.

If you can do three sets of fifteen, try to increase the number of repetitions per set and attempt to do your pushups faster.

(If your wrists hurt when performing the move, instead of placing your hands on the floor, hold on to dumbbells, which reduces the pressure on small wrist joints.)

(continued)

The Modified Pushup

Kneel on the floor, placing the hands on the floor shoulder width apart in front of you. Lower your upper body to the floor, keeping your back straight during the movement. Lower your upper body from the kneeling position. When you can do three sets of fifteen, attempt the Traditional, Basic Pushup.

Incline Pushup

Stabilizing yourself from a low bookcase, table, chair, or sofa, and keeping your feet together, hands shoulder width apart, push your body off to arms' length. Lower your upper body to the support, then push off again. When you can do three sets of fifteen, either use a lower support (a stabilized lower chair or table) or move on to the Modified Pushup.

Wall Pushoff

While standing with your feet together, hands against the wall, shoulder width apart, lean into the wall and push off from this position. Lower your upper body to the wall and push off from here. If this is too easy, try taking a large step back and do the movement at an incline. When you can do a full routine of three sets of fifteen, move on to the Incline Pushup.

Flat Bench Dumbbell Chest Presses

Primary muscle group worked: Pectorals (chest).

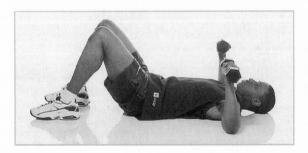

Lie on the floor or a bench with a dumbbell in each hand. Your feet should either be flat on the floor or up on the bench with your knees bent, depending upon which position is more comfortable.

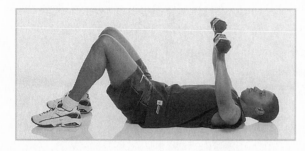

Starting with the dumbbells slightly to your side and parallel to your chest, exhale and push the weights upward in a pyramid motion until your arms are directly above your shoulders and your palms are facing upward. Keep your back flat against the bench.

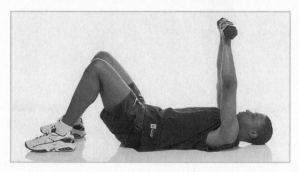

Slowly lower the weights until your elbows are slightly below your shoulders.

One-Arm Dumbbell Rows

Primary muscle group worked: Latissimus dorsi (back).

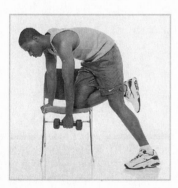
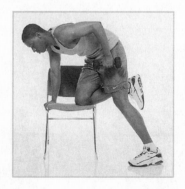

Kneel with your left hand and knee on your weight bench and your right foot flat on the floor. Hold a dumbbell in your right hand, keeping your neck, back, and shoulders parallel to the floor, your abdominal muscles pulled in and firm. Let your arm hang down naturally, palm inward toward your body and knuckles pointed toward the floor as you grip the weight. Pull the dumbbell upward, squeezing the middle back, as if you are starting a lawn mower. Don't forget to keep your back flat. Pull until your upper arm is parallel to the floor and your hand is even with your waist. Slowly lower weight to starting position. Do all the repetitions for one arm before switching to the opposite arm.

Barbell Good Mornings

Primary muscle group worked: Latissimus dorsi (back).

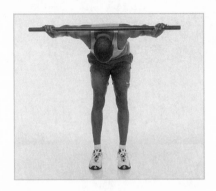

Stand erect with your feet together and knees slightly bent (don't let them lock out). Hold an exercise bar behind your neck with your hands slightly wider than shoulder width. Don't rest the bar on your shoulders; support it with your hands. Slowly bend forward at the waist until your upper body is parallel to the floor. Exhale and come up slowly to the starting position, keeping your back flat and head centered.

Dumbbell Side Laterals

Primary muscle group worked: Deltoids (shoulders).

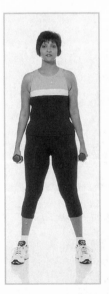
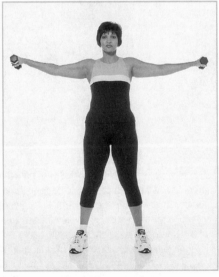

These can be performed seated or standing. Sit up straight with feet shoulder width apart. Hold dumbbells in each hand with arms slightly away from your sides, palms turned toward your thighs. Exhale and raise the dumbbells shoulder high, leading with your elbows. Slowly lower the weights. At bottom of the movement, hold the dumbbells slightly away from your sides.

Seated Dumbbell Presses

Primary muscle group worked: Deltoids (shoulders).

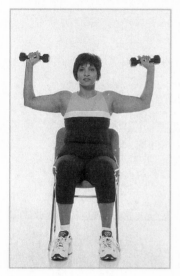 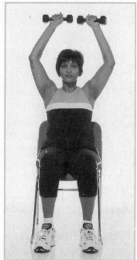

Sit with feet shoulder width apart and body erect. Raise dumbbells to your shoulders with your palms facing forward and arms bent to a ninety-degree angle. Visualize a pyramid and concentrate on pressing the weight up its sides. Exhale and press dumbbells overhead at this angle until your elbows are nearly locked, but not quite. Avoid banging the weights at the peak of the pyramid. Slowly lower the weights.

Alternate Dumbbell Curls

Primary muscle group worked: Biceps (front of upper arm).

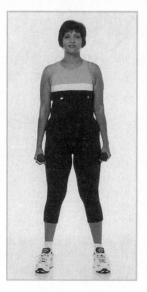 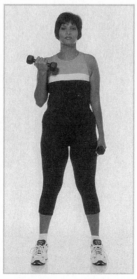

These can be performed seated or standing. Hold a pair of dumbbells with your arms at your sides, palms facing your thighs. Exhale and twist as you lift one dumbbell—elbows close to your side—turning your palm up and slowly curling up to your shoulder. As you curl each arm upward, make sure to keep your wrists parallel with your forearms. Lower your arm to the starting position, then alternate with your other arm.

Dumbbell Biceps Curls

Primary muscle group worked: Biceps (front of upper arm).

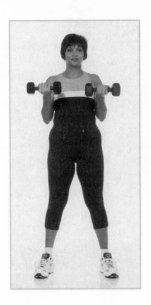

Stand with your feet shoulder width apart, a dumbbell in each hand. Let your arms hang down at your sides with your palms pointed away from your body. Keeping your elbows tight to your body, curl both arms upward and really squeeze your biceps until the weights are in front of your shoulders. Slowly lower the dumbbells to the starting position.

Dumbbell Seated Overhead Extensions

Primary muscle group worked: Triceps (back of upper arm).

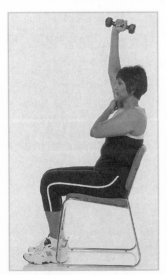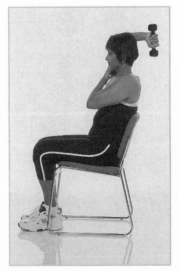

Holding a dumbbell in one hand, fully extend your arm over your head. Support your upper arm with the opposite hand, then slowly lower the dumbbell behind your head as if to scratch your back. Exhale and extend your arm to the starting position. Complete the set. Repeat with your opposite arm.

Bench Dips

Primary muscle group worked: Triceps (back of upper arm).

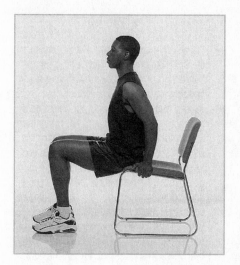
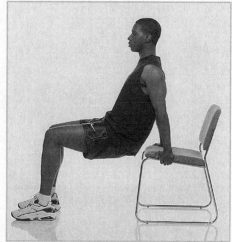

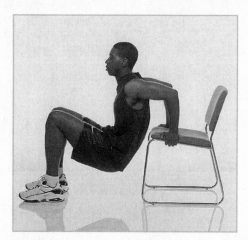

Sit on the edge of a bench. With your arms straight at your sides, place your hands palms-down and grip the edge of the bench. Take two or three steps forward and away from the bench, then lower your body until your arms are bent at a 90-degree angle. Exhale and push back to starting position. Squeeze your triceps at top position. Note: To maximize the use of your arms rather than your torso, squeeze your triceps as you push up.

Lower-Body Exercises

Squats

Primary muscle group worked: Quadriceps (front of thigh).

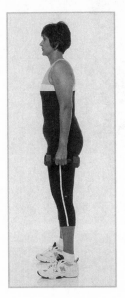
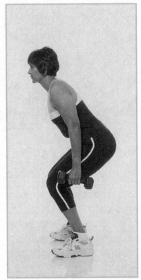

These are the most popular leg exercise because they're known for building shapely thighs and buttocks. Stand with your feet shoulder width apart with your weight resting slightly backward toward your heels. Hold dumbbells at your side or, if you're not ready for dumbbells, rest your hands on your hips. Slowly lower your body as if to sit in a chair, keeping your back straight and taking care not to let your heels lift off the floor. Lower your body as far as you can without leaning your body more than a few inches forward. Lower yourself until your thighs are horizontal to the floor, but no farther. Also make sure that your knees don't jut out beyond your toes. Once you feel your upper body begin to lean forward over your thighs, straighten your legs and push upward with your thighs to the starting position.

Lunges

Primary muscle group worked: Hamstrings (back of thigh).

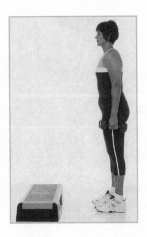
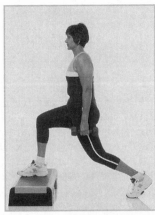

Perhaps the most effective exercise for firming and toning the muscles in the back of your legs and your buttocks, lunges also strengthen the front of the thighs (quadriceps). Stand with your feet together, chest up, and shoulders back, approximately two feet from a block or step. Hold one dumbbell in each hand with your palms facing inward, toward your legs. Take a long step forward onto the step. Keeping your back straight, bend your front knee over the ball of your foot until your thigh is horizontal; your back knee should be slightly bent. Exhale and push back to starting position. Switch legs. For maximum effect, keep your back straight and leg motion slow and deliberate.

Stiff-Leg Dead Lifts

Primary muscle group worked: Hamstrings (back of thigh).

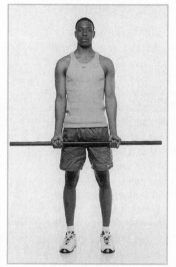
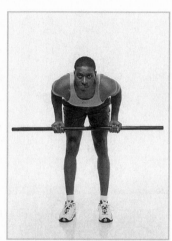

This exercise will add shape and fullness to the rear thigh area. Rest a barbell in your hands (your hands should be underneath the bar) at thigh level, while standing erect, feet shoulder width apart. Bend forward until your back is flat and head neutral. Keep your knees locked. Exhale and let your head lead your body back into an upright position.

Standing Toe Raises

Primary muscle group worked: Calves.

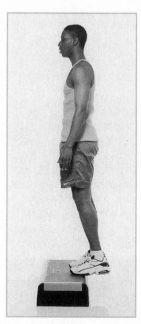
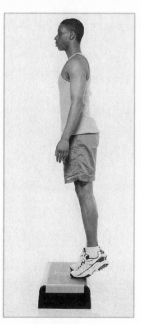

Stand on the edge of a step with the balls of your feet firmly upon the step, heels hanging off. For balance, lightly hold on to the stair rail, a wall, or another object. Lower your heels below the step, feeling your calf muscles stretch. Then push up slowly until you're standing on your tiptoes or as high as your leg will extend. Return to the starting position. Note: Don't neglect your calves on leg day. Fully developed calves anchor the feet during squats and aid in balance.

Abdominal Exercises

Bent-Knee Crunches

Primary muscle group worked: Upper abdominals.

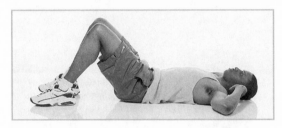

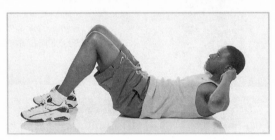

Lie on your back in a bent-knee sit-up position, feet shoulder width apart. To avoid pulling on the back of your neck, place your fingertips behind your ear lobes or on your temples, with your elbows pointed outward. Using your abdominal muscles, slowly curl up and forward until you raise your shoulders off the floor. Slowly return to the starting position.

Feet-Up Crunches

Primary muscle group worked: Lower abdominals.

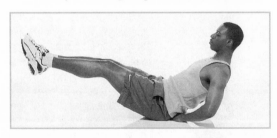

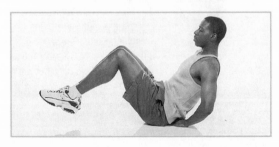

Holding your hands near your behind to help you balance, rest on your tailbone with your feet about six inches above the floor. Keep your legs together and draw your knees up toward your chest. Contract your lower abdominal muscles and repeatedly move your upper and lower body closer together in a short range of motion without letting your feet touch the floor.

Think It Through

There's a direct connection between physical and mental power. Lifting weights requires strength, focus, and determination. There will be many times your muscles will be so tired you'll want to drop the weight and quit. But if you push one more time, you may be surprised to find that you can actually do the repetition.

Sometimes pushing past the point where you previously failed gives us confidence in our ability to overcome other obstacles. Other times, it just feels great to experience the benefits of being physically stronger— being able to carry a couple of children, armloads of groceries, or two bulky suitcases up a flight of stairs.

But these qualities—strength, focus, self-confidence, and determination—can be applied to the rest of our lives and are particularly useful when we're breaking bad habits and replacing them with new ones. As you gain confidence by lifting weights, apply those characteristics to another aspect of your challenge. Notice how the sense of being in control of a physical challenge can help you master a mental one. Tap into your newly discovered willpower next time you walk through the supermarket and smell fried chicken in the prepared-foods section. Exercise discipline by sticking to your calorie count for the day. Practice determination by walking up and down the stairs instead of taking the elevator. In your Food and Fitness Diary, make a list of ten things related to losing weight that require any of these characteristics.

For Your Spirit

By now your body's probably feeling at least a little sore and achy. What a great time to take a relaxing aromatherapy bath. If you don't already have aromatic bathsalts, you can go out and purchase some, or you can make your own, inexpensively at home.

To make your own aromatherapy salts, pick up some sea salt and baking soda or Epsom salts on your next visit to your local pharmacy or health-food store. Sea salt detoxifies the body and conditions your skin. Baking soda and Epsom salts help to soothe aching muscles. Combine the sea salt with one of the other two salts and add ¼ cup of this mixture to your bath, followed by 10 to 15 drops of your favorite essential oil. (Essential oils can be purchased at many health-food stores, as well as at most popular bath and body shops.) Chamomile, eucalyptus, geranium, jasmine, lavender, lilac, lily of the valley, orange, vanilla, and ylang-ylang are all relaxing and can create a feeling of well-being and balance.

Combine sea salt and baking soda in your bath with eucalyptus, lavender, and rosemary oils to make a fragrant bath that relieves achy joints (rosemary helps relieve achy muscles). Or combine lavender with orange oil to create a more relaxing aroma.

Draw some warm water into your bathtub, turn on some quiet, relaxing music, turn off the phone, and tell your family that you love them, but to leave you alone. Now's your time to chill and give thanks for the willpower to make healthy lifestyle changes.

CHAPTER 12

Putting It All Together Now

The *HealthQuest* Workouts

When it comes to exercise, certified fitness trainer Charsie Herndon of Atlanta says, "Results are invariably measured by how much, how often, and how long you work out." The more devoted you are to your workout, the more quickly you'll speed up your metabolism, the faster you'll override your body's instinct to conserve calories, and the more dramatic the changes you'll notice in your body, mind, and spirit. As a result, if you're at least holding your calories constant, the more rapidly you're going to lose weight.

By now, you probably have a good idea of how to reduce the number of calories you eat, but you may find that trying to figure out how to juggle stretching, strength training, and aerobic exercise is more than just a notion. So we're going to help you by pulling it all together. This chapter contains a 7-day workout routine that combines all three aspects of physical fitness to help you lose weight at the maximum rate. We suggest that you make this routine (or one that's similar to it) the core exercise regimen of your *HealthQuest* 30-Day Weight-Loss Program.

But we also provide you with an easier starter program—one that you can do at home, costs nothing, and needs no special equipment. It's simple, uses all your major muscle groups, will get your body moving and your heart rate up, and in no time will give you the results you need to keep you motivated. The only thing required for this workout is your own body, so we've named this our *HealthQuest* No Excuses Workout. We're sure once you start it, you'll look forward to your daily workouts and appreciate the way your body looks and feels and the awareness of your newly toned muscles.

The Split Routine

The strength-training portion of this regimen is a *split-routine work-out*. You train some of your muscles during one workout and train others a day or two later, but you never strength train your whole body in one session. In addition to the three days of strength-training exercises, this program includes five days of stretching, four days of abdominal work, and three days of aerobic exercise. To give your body a rest, we've planned for two days off.

Depending upon how vigorously you want to work out, it will take you between thirty and ninety minutes to complete the exercises each day. Because the content of the program varies, some days the workout will take longer to complete than other days. If you're strapped for time, you can finish the workout more quickly by completing the lowest number of sets recommended for each exercise and working out aerobically for the shorter duration. The entire program can be done at home or at your gym, using free weights or weight machines.

We told you that the workout is divided over several days. Well, there are several ways to split a strength-training routine. We're going to focus on an upper- and lower-body split routine. In this workout, you'll strength train your upper body during one session, followed by your lower body and small muscle groups during the next workout.

Now, don't forget, our objective is to expend 250 calories each day by exercising. To maximize the number of calories you burn, stick to the basics of each movement, concentrate on feeling your muscles work, and maintain a steady rhythm. Don't forget to exhale as you push or pull the weight during the resistance phase, and inhale as you release. Don't lift too much weight or do too many reps or sets; it will impede your progress. Most of all, appreciate yourself and your body while you do the routine.

The Upper/Lower Body Split-Routine Workout

Day 1 • CHEST AND BACK

Exercise	Sets	Reps
Warm-Up		
5–7 minute brisk walk		
Stretch		
3–5 minutes		
Chest		
Flat-Bench Dumbbell Flys (page 192)	2	12
Flat-Bench Dumbbell Chest Presses (page 194)	2–3	12
Back		
Barbell Good Mornings (page 196)	2–3	12
One-Arm Dumbbell Rows (page 195)	2–3	12
Abs		
Bent-Knee Crunches (page 202)	2–3	20–25
Feet-Up Crunches (page 202)	2–3	20–25
Aerobics		
Brisk walk, jog, low-impact aerobics		
20–30 minutes		
Cool Down		
5 minutes		
Stretch/Deep Breathing		
5 minutes		

Day 2 • LEGS AND TRICEPS

Exercise	Sets	Reps
Warm-Up		
5–7 minute brisk walk		
Stretch		
3–5 minutes		
Legs		
Squats (page 200)	2	12
Lunges (page 200)	2–3	12–15
Stiff-Leg Dead Lifts (page 201)	2–3	12
Standing Toe Raises (page 201)	2–3	15–20
Triceps		
Dumbbell Seated Overhead Extensions (page 198)	2–3	12
Bench Dips (page 199)	2–3	12
Aerobics		
Brisk walk, jog, low-impact aerobics		
20–30 minutes		
Cool Down		
5 minutes		
Stretch/Deep Breathing		
Quads, Hamstring, Calves		
5 minutes		

Day 3 • AEROBICS, ABS, STRETCHING

After two consecutive sessions of strengthening workouts, it is time to let the muscles rest and recover, and give the body a chance to respond to what it has been through. The focus today is on aerobics, abs, and stretching. Don't hesitate to elect a gentle aerobic method, like walking, to ease you into the program.

Aerobics
20–45 minutes

Abs

Bent-Knee Crunches (page 202)	2–3	20–25
Feet-Up Crunches (page 202)	2–3	20–25

Stretching
Minimum 5 minutes

Day 4 • REST

Productive use of quiet time is the best reward for rest day. Get a minimum 5 to 10 minutes of time to yourself with no distractions. Protect your entire workout time if at all possible.

Day 5 • SHOULDERS AND BICEPS

Exercise	Sets	Reps
Warm-Up		
5–7 minute brisk walk		
Stretch		
3–5 minutes		
Shoulders		
Dumbbell Side Laterals (page 196)	2–3	12
Seated Dumbbell Presses (page 197)	2–3	12
Biceps		
Dumbbell Bicep Curls (standing) (page 198)	2–3	12
Alternate Dumbbell Curls (seated) (page 197)	2–3	12
Abs		
Bent-Knee Crunches (page 202)	2–3	20–25
Feet-Up Crunches (page 202)	2–3	20–25
Aerobics		
Brisk walk, jog, low-impact aerobics 20–30 minutes		
Cool Down		
5 minutes		
Stretch/Deep Breathing		
5 minutes		

Day 6 • AEROBICS, ABS, STRETCHING

Aerobics

20–45 minutes

Abs

Brisk walk, jog, low-impact aerobics

Stretching

Minimum 5 minutes

Day 7 • REST

It's time to tally the past few days on a mind-body-spirit note. Pull away and just chill.

The *HealthQuest* No-Excuses Workout

This workout is a simple full-body routine of toning exercises that uses your own body weight. If you are new to exercise and haven't exercised much before, this workout is a good way to get started. You won't need any special equipment except a sturdy chair. Unlike the split routine, this exercise circuit works your entire body in the same session. You'll work all your major muscle groups three times a week, finishing each workout with moderate aerobics and abdominal work. You'll do a longer session of aerobics and stretching on two additional days, and be off for two days. The exercises are explained on pages 192–202.

The Full-Body Workout

Days 1, 3, 5 •

Exercise	Sets	Reps
Warm-Up		
5–7 minute brisk walk		
Stretch		
3–5 minutes		
Upper Body		
Pushup (or Pushoffs) (page 193)	2–3	15–20
Bicep Curls (no weight) (page 198)	2–3	15–20
Tricep Bench Dips (page 199)	2–3	15–20
Lower Body		
Squats (page 200)	2	12
Lunges (page 200)	2–3	12–15
Standing Toe Raises (page 201)	2–3	15–20
Abs		
Bent-Knee Crunches (page 202)	2–3	20–25
Feet-Up Crunches (page 202)	2–3	20–25
Aerobics		
Brisk walk, jog, low-impact aerobics		
20 minutes		

Cool Down
5 minutes

Stretch/Deep Breathing
5 minutes

Days 2 and 4 •

Warm-Up
5–7 minute brisk walk

Stretch
3–5 minutes

Aerobics
Brisk walk, jog, low-impact aerobics
30–40 minutes

Cool Down
5 minutes

Stretch/Deep Breathing
5 minutes

Days 6 and 7 •

After five consecutive sessions of workouts, let your muscles rest and recover. If you're up for it, undertake a walk or other gentle, fun activity that you enjoy and keeps you moving. You can also do your stretching routine for relaxation and to keep you limber.

How Much Exercise?

How do you know if you're overdoing your workouts? And how do you know if you're not pushing yourself hard enough? Here are some signs to keep an eye out for:

Signs and Symptoms of Overtraining

- Chronic muscle or joint soreness.
- Training same body parts two days in a row.
- An attitude that exercise is good, so more is better. Wrong! Don't go there.
- Increased resting heart rate.
- Increased resting blood pressure.
- Insomnia, indigestion, lack of appetite.
- Decreased endurance, increased fatigue.
- Anxiety, irritability, depression.
- Increased incidence of injuries.
- Increased incidence of colds and infections.
- Strenuous workouts more than three consecutive days.

Signs and Symptoms of Undertraining

- Loss of intensity from existing level.
- Loss in strength and endurance.
- Resting more than three consecutive days between workouts.
- Taking too much time between sets (more than 3 to 4 minutes).
- Lifting same weight forever (longer than 4 to 6 months).
- Doing unstructured hit-and-miss workouts (by rushing or by not having a plan).
- Repetitive use of improper technique.
- Lack of mind-body-spirit connection during workouts.
- Overly engaging in distractions and interruptions (talking during sets, blasting headphones, etc.).

Think It Through

Let's return to the subject of obstacles. By now perhaps you've bought new sneakers and have joined a gym. You did the exercises in chapter 9 to identify and overcome the obstacles you'd face to becoming active. You thought that by doing these things, you'd feel more motivated and exercising would be easier—or at least somewhat enjoyable. But now you've actually been trying to do the workouts we've provided. Not only are you encountering the obstacles you identified in chapter 9, now you're thinking of new ones: *My body is sore and it hurts. . . . I don't like how it feels when I'm breathing so hard. . . . There's only one other person my size in my dance class. . . .* Your thoughts may even be starting to snowball.

You start with one negative thought and it mushrooms into several others. *I can't do this working-out thing. Now I'll only lose weight at half the rate I had planned to. That means it's going to take me twice as long. I'll be doing this forever. I knew it wasn't going to work!*

But have you ever noticed how negative thinking snowballs, while positive thinking doesn't? When was the last time you took something positive and built on it? It's been a while, hasn't it? Maybe this is a good time to change that. *I made it through two aerobics classes this week. It was hard, but if I made it through two this week, then I can make it through two next week. In just a couple weeks, I should be able to handle three. After that, maybe I'll start to lift weights once a week. Then I'll really be losing weight fast. I'll be well on my way. Plus, by then, I'll probably be enjoying it. If I'm enjoying it, maybe I'll continue to exercise even after I've lost the weight. Wow, I feel like I'll actually be able to keep it off this time! Boy, this isn't as hard as I thought it would be. . . .*

For Your Spirit

The biggest obstacle to success is often our Self. All the chatter taking place inside your head—the internal dialogue telling you why this will never work—is merely an old part of yourself that's afraid of dying off. It will battle the new you. As a matter of fact, you may literally feel at war with your old habits. The old you may not leave without kicking and screaming. It may try to hold on until it's last breath.

Ready to kick the old you to the curb so you can start to embrace the new? Every time you notice yourself engaging in negative thoughts or speaking of things in negative language (like, *I can't do whatever. . . . It won't work. . . . It will never happen. . . . etc.*), flip the script and say it in a positive and affirming way, as you learned how to do when you made positive affirmations back in chapter 2.

Let's give the old you a run for the money. Turn back to page 26 now and review the section on affirmations. Go ahead, do it right now!

Now pick three negative things you've been saying to yourself about exercising. Write them in your Food and Fitness Diary.

Now look at them in a positive light. Rather than focusing on what you can't do, try building on the progress you've made so far. Then let it snowball like in the example above. Write in your Food and Fitness Diary and really let it rip. Keep writing until you've turned all your negative internal chatter into an exciting and positive future.

Now, remembering the power of the spoken word, state these positive possibilities out loud. Notice how you feel about yourself as you give voice to your hopes and dreams for your future. You may feel your mood become more positive, your attitude become lighter, your energy increase. You may even find yourself feeling motivated to go exercise right now.

Keep the positive vibes alive by starting to act out of this new energy. Next time you feel yourself starting to grind to a halt, repeat this exercise and ride the vibes for as long as they'll take you. We guarantee that you'll end up in a new place.

CHAPTER 13

Keeping It Real

What to Do When
the Clouds Roll In

The pounds are starting to melt away. You've traded your after-noon pastry for fresh fruit salad, added a three-mile walk into your daily routine, and begun to meditate to keep your nerves calm—and you're reaping the rich benefits of your new health-oriented lifestyle. Then one day you weigh yourself and realize the needle's in the same place it was a week ago. Another week goes by, and still no change. Or maybe the weight is coming off, but the exercise every day is getting to be a drag.

Creating a new and improved you isn't always smooth sailing. The pounds might not come tumbling off as you want them to. Or you might lose weight for a while, then reach a plateau. You might even be tempted to try drastic measures when these disappointments hit home. But the keys to maintaining your weight loss and your healthy diet is to stay com-mitted and to realize that, if you start to get frustrated with the process, you're not alone.

"I was an impulsive eater, and the stuff I ate was terrible for my body," A.J. says. "Sometimes after dinner I used to drive over to McDonald's and mow through a Big Mac and fries like they were an after-dinner mint."

But over the course of several months, she had begun to come to terms with her eating habits, which she admitted were out of control. And she had been sailing along on her weight-loss plan. So when she hit the wall, she felt like an utter failure.

Meditation helped bring A.J. a measure of inner peace that in turn helped her identify two abusive men in her life—her boss and her boyfriend—as the source of the anxiety she salved by overeating. As she took steps to change her relationship with them, she also was able to redefine her relationship with food and to improve her attitude toward exercise. She substituted baked potatoes for fries and lean beef for burgers, and then gradually began an early morning walking routine. Sure enough, the miracle began: before she even realized it, A.J. was losing nearly two pounds a week.

"It was like magic," she recalls, beaming at the accomplishment.

But the magic was short-lived. Twenty-five pounds later, her weight loss gradually came to a halt, despite her continued walking and healthful eating. And no matter how hard A.J. tried, she couldn't shake the chunkiness around her hips.

"I really did feel that I had failed, although I couldn't figure out where," says A.J. "I wasn't doing anything differently than before, but still the weight wasn't going anywhere. Talk about feeling down!"

A.J.'s frustration is more common than she probably realized. Many people who manage to lose weight feel disappointment and even despair when their early successes seem to wither. Some feel tempted to resort to extreme measures, starving themselves in an attempt to keep the pounds coming off.

But there are good reasons to be patient with yourself if your weight loss doesn't match your expectations. The body is superintelligent, created with all kinds of self-correcting mechanisms. If it wants dust out of your nose, you sneeze. If a hair flies in your eye, tears rush to wash it away. Even chills and choking serve a useful purpose in getting the body back to equilibrium. Your metabolism is no different. It's there to help you keep on enough weight to survive.

We know, we know—you've got enough pounds to save yourself and a couple other folks, too. Still, there are excellent reasons not to resort to drastic measures to try to force the process along. Let's talk about some of the common frustrations—and the biological and psychological factors behind them—that can creep into even the most stellar weight-loss plan and what you can do about them.

I can lose weight, but not from the right places.

That's one of the most common weight-loss dilemmas. It typically affects women who find that they can lose weight from their belly and breasts but not their hips and thighs. The issue here is basic biology. Remember the discussion of "apples" and "pears" in chapter 6? Men tend to be more apples: They tend to concentrate their extra fat in their bellies, where it is easily retrieved when they need energy. On the other hand, women are more often pears, with more fat in their hips and thighs. This lower-body fat is the result of divine design: It cushions and protects a woman's reproductive organs and is used during pregnancy and nursing to provide calories for a growing infant. That's why nursing women often lose their pregnancy weight faster than those who bottle-feed. If you're not pregnant or nursing, it can be awfully hard to get rid of fat from that part of your body. That's why women who embark on excellent exercise and eating plans often find that they lose weight from their face, their breasts, their stomach—everywhere but their hips and thighs.

Experiences like this remind us that, while we may want to fit into a really nice pair of pants or that certain skimpy swimsuit, our bodies have a job to do—and being too thin may not be among the job requirements. Human beings have a larger purpose: to help propagate the species. So as much as we'd like to think we're in complete control of our destiny, we are all born with genetic instructions that help ensure that whatever else we do, we pass on life to the next generation.

Does this mean it's fruitless to even try to lose weight? Not at all. First, revisit your exercise routine. If you're trying to get rid of your belly but you aren't doing any ab work, that could be one of your problems right there. Focus your attention on the areas that most need it. The same is true with your thighs. Add some leg exercises to your routine. Sign up for an aerobics class; we guarantee you'll work your hips and thighs.

But when you know you've done your very disciplined best, you shouldn't blame yourself if you can't seem to lose weight from the "right" places. It also means that when it comes to setting weight-loss goals, it makes sense to be flexible and forgiving. If your body seems reluctant to achieve the shape you envision, maybe it's your ideal body *image* that needs reshaping so that it falls more in line with what your body is capable of achieving.

I've always been big, and I can't seem to lose the mega-pounds I want.

You can change your weight to a degree, especially if your extra pounds come from being misnourished (like too many calories coming from fat), overeating (like there's no tomorrow), or from putting off exercising (as if tomorrow is all there is). If your waistline comes primarily from your lifestyle, changing one should change the other.

But at least a portion of your body size is inherited from Mom and Dad. So, if you eat well and you're reasonably active, but you come from a big family, then there may be limits to how radically you can change your size. If you inherited big hips, even the strictest adherence to the *HealthQuest* 30-Day Weight-Loss Program won't make you a waif. In that sense, changing your weight can be a little like altering your height.

Which is not to say all is lost. First of all, your diet and exercise program will help you get into the healthiest, fittest shape possible. Then, too, you have to remember that you are not your weight. Your body size doesn't define who you are any more than your sock size. That can be difficult to accept when you're immersed in a world that awards people status based on the strangest criteria (skin color, for one). But it's true. If you have trouble accepting yourself as you are, regardless of your weight, the meditation exercises in this book can deliver you a sense of centeredness and peace of mind that can help.

I lost weight for a while, but now I've hit a plateau and I can't seem to lose an ounce.

Nutritionists theorize that everyone's metabolism is programmed to function at a certain rate—that "set point" we talked about earlier—that your body likes to maintain. When you lose many pounds early in a diet, only to see your losses trail off until they eventually stop completely, your set point may have been called into action.

Remember that when you lose a lot of weight, your body thinks you're starving, so your set point adjusts to a lower level so you burn fewer calories. (Your body also flips your hunger switch so that you go after more food.) Repeated periods of calorie deprivation drive your set point lower and lower, which is why yo-yo dieting—on this week, off the next—is ultimately counterproductive. But when you eat a nutritious, balanced diet, you can lose weight without disturbing your set point.

If you've lost weight but find that your progress has slowed, you may be eating too *little*, particularly too few carbohydrates. That sounds odd— how could eating more cause you to lose more weight? But it's true. A higher-carb diet revs your metabolism, so that as long as you go easy on your fat intake, you should burn off more pounds—and continue to do so without hitting a plateau. So make sure you're eating plenty of whole grains, fruits, and vegetables that are prepared the heart-healthy, low-fat way. That's **Step #1**.

Step #2: Take a hard look at your activity level. Has it changed over time? Once you start losing weight, it's easy to take for granted whatever you did to get there. If walking for an hour every evening after dinner worked for you, it's only natural after a while to relax. You might figure to yourself, *"I can walk for half an hour, get back in time to catch Oprah, and still lose weight!"* If you're losing as a result of a certain amount of exercise, definitely don't do less. If you stop losing weight, it could be a sign that you need to return to whatever exercise level got you on track in the first place. Also, make sure you're being honest with yourself about how much you're working out. Just as we tend to *underestimate* the amount of food we eat, we tend to *overestimate* the amount of time we spend working out.

How much exercise do you have to do to keep the weight off? When researchers at the University of Wisconsin studied formerly obese women who had lost as many as fifty pounds, they found that the women who exercised moderately for eighty minutes a day, or those who exercised more intensely for thirty-five minutes a day, had regained an average of only six pounds a year later. Your best bet: Make sure you've reached your target weight before you ease up on the duration and/or intensity of your workouts.

I was really pumped when I started my *HealthQuest* 30-Day Weight-Loss Program, but now I don't feel as motivated.

It's normal to experience letdowns now and then—times when it's difficult to rev yourself up to stick with your program. Sometimes, the most nutrition-minded diner can slip up in a Mississippi Mud Pie, and the most spiritual person can find meditating mundane. The most disciplined exerciser might wake up one morning and roll over instead of doing crunches. Even elite athletes experience periods when they just can't seem to summon their usual motivation.

If this happens to you, remember to take one day at a time. The fact that it may be difficult to stick with your program today doesn't mean you'll feel the same way tomorrow. Even if you've fallen off the wagon for a month, don't give up, assuming your situation will remain unchanged for the next month.

Ask yourself why you feel stuck and look for creative ways to keep your groove from becoming a rut. Have elements of your fitness routine become, well, routine? At first it might seem as though your body will never become accustomed to the new paces you're putting it through. But it will. And then it will get bored with the same old, same old. So mix it up. If you're a walker, runner, or hiker, vary your route, your distance, or your pace. If you swim, add a water aerobics class to your regular laps. If you bike—a lower-body workout—do some upper-body work, too. One of the great benefits of cross-training—besides its ability to work different sets of muscles and thus provide a balanced workout—is that variety helps maintain your interest.

The same goes for what you eat. If you find yourself looking at your plate and muttering *Been there, done that* maybe it's time to revamp your diet. Experiment with more of the recipes we've provided in the back of the book. Treat yourself to a low-fat cookbook and pick up some new menu ideas. Visit your supermarket or natural foods store and check out a vegetable, fruit, or grain you've never tried before.

What about your spiritual side? If you suddenly find it difficult to keep your mind on living mindfully, think about what could be influencing your lack of attention to or interest in that part of your life. Has your life suddenly gotten busier, crazier, more hectic? Are your meditations uninspired? You may have simply strayed away from some of the key principles that help enrich your spiritual center. Try putting a little more effort into enhancing your spiritual side. Treat yourself to a minirefresher course by reviewing the spiritual exercises in this book, or try a new church, mosque, or other place of worship. Now could be the time when you need a stronger spiritual grounding.

In all aspects of this weight-loss program—and your whole life, for that matter—start fresh each day and renew your commitment to yourself. Remind yourself of why you started your *HealthQuest* 30-Day Weight-Loss Program, and remember that yesterday is a done deal: You can't change it; all you can do is to learn from it.

Moving Down the Road

• Whether your first thirty days are glass-smooth or a bit bumpier than you expected, keep your weight-loss plan in perspective.

• It's perfectly healthy to gaze into the mirror and imagine a new you, but remember there's no such thing as a perfect body. Set reasonable goals for yourself; if you wear size 20 don't try to force your way down to a size 2. That way, you help protect yourself against going overboard and having your weight-loss plan develop into an obsession—as well as the devastation that comes when you realize you've set yourself up to fail. Give yourself a break. If perfection is impossible, why chase it? Then again, if you believe that God created us in the image of divinity, then maybe you're fine just the way you are.

• Think of weight loss as part of a larger journey toward wholeness. After all, if losing weight were about nothing but getting rid of a mess of fat cells, you could take your VISA card to the nearest plastic surgeon and get them sucked away. It's infinitely preferable to view weight loss as part of a larger effort to be healthy, content with yourself, and at peace with the universe. When you do this, you view losing weight as a means to an end—and a wonderful one at that—rather than as an end in itself. That end is a life in which you're healthy, fit, and happy with yourself all the way around.

- And most of all, make sure you're losing weight for the right reasons. It's one thing to embark on a weight-loss plan to feel healthier, or lighter on your feet, or more comfortable in your body. It's quite another to lose weight because you think it will help you catch a mate, or because you're tired of your parents nagging you, or your friends teasing you about your size, or because you want the boss to pay more attention to you. In other words, lose weight for yourself—not someone else.

Think It Through

At regular intervals during your program, take a quiet moment to sit down with your diary and assess the progress you're making toward your goals. Review your original goals. Ask yourself the following questions and jot the answers in your diary. Really delve deeply into any one that seems to need your attention. (You'll know which ones they are because of the funny feeling you get in the pit of your stomach when you answer.)

- Are my goals the same as they were when I started? (Remember: Things change—including our goals.)
- Am I keeping to my fitness/workout goal? If not, why? Do I need to adjust it? How?
- Am I keeping to my eating goal? If not, why? Do I need to adjust it? How?
- What can I do to spice up my routine?
- What have I learned about myself during this process?
- What changes have I seen in myself—in my body, my mind, and my spirit—since I began the program?

For Your Spirit

Turn to chapter 2 and find the self-love affirmations. Repeat them, then repeat them again until the words begin to hum inside you. This is the creative energy that you'll need to really rely on as you move through each set of thirty days and to incorporate these changes into a new lifestyle.

CHAPTER 14

Keep On Keepin' On

Going It Alone

Congratulations! You've done something many people just dream about—you've jump-started a successful journey to permanent weight loss and total wellness. You're changing old, unhealthy habits. You feel emotionally and spiritually vibrant and energetic. You're happier with the way your body looks and feels. Be very, very proud of this accomplishment.

But it's not over. Your new, healthy eating, exercise, and spiritual habits are a lifestyle change, remember? And depending upon your weight-loss goals, you may want to start another set of thirty days—and maybe another and another. If so, take a day to celebrate your success. Reward yourself with something you've been wanting to do: purchase a new outfit to fit your more slender figure or new equipment for your home gym, indulge in a relaxing day at the spa, go to the game or to see your favorite performer in concert, treat yourself to a play or a comedy show. Just make sure to do something special to celebrate reaching this important milestone. After all, you're the star in your own show—and stardom has its perks and rewards. Afterward, gather yourself, create a new set of goals for the next thirty days, ask God for strength, then start again.

Or maybe you've reached your weight-loss goal. If so, give yourself a hand! You, too, should reward yourself, then hunker down to maintain the good habits that got you this far. The thing about weight loss isn't losing the weight, but keeping it off. And what's the point of such a healthy accomplishment if you can't enjoy it indefinitely. That means not just being able to look at a bathroom scale and smile; it also means maintaining a healthy emotional state and a positive spiritual balance.

In the previous chapter, you learned what to do when your weight-loss plans hit a snag. But even if you don't encounter big-time obstacles, you'll need to know how to keep a good thing going. Here's some advice that will help you sustain indefinitely the terrific new habits you're learning.

Remember: You're in control.

When you commit yourself to a new way of living, it's only natural to try to conform to all the rules and guidelines, reading and heeding the fine print, so to speak. That's good; you want to be squarely onboard the program. But remember that your *HealthQuest* 30-Day Weight-Loss Program isn't controlling you; you control it. You decide how fast to move through the program, what direction to take it, what goals you want to meet, and when you've met those goals. If you want to lose more weight, just repeat the program in thirty-day increments until you've reached the weight you want.

When you remember who's in control, you're less likely to be hard on yourself when something unexpected happens. If you splurge and mow through half of a thick-crust pizza for dinner when you know that's not on your diet plan, just resolve to forgo dessert that night and get back on track tomorrow. That's a lot healthier than feeling that you're a failure because you haven't measured up to the rules of the program. You're in charge.

Be ever mindful of what, when, and how much you eat.

You've learned the principles of mindful eating. But like any new skill, it takes practice to make it a part of your life. So keep using mealtimes as an opportunity for increasing awareness—mental, physical, and spiritual. Check yourself periodically to make sure you're fully aware of:

- *What* you're eating. Is it compatible with your goals for weight loss and healthy eating, or has it snuck onto your plate unawares?

- *When* you're eating. Is the timing in concert with your own natural feelings of hunger, or are you eating when it's convenient or when you're nervous about something?

• *How much* you're eating. Are you eating just enough to satisfy your body's needs, or are you overdoing it?

One of the easiest ways to make sure you don't overeat is to *slow down*. If your life is frenzied, use mealtimes to decompress, to truly enjoy your meal, whether solo or with friends or family, so that you leave the table moving at a more human tempo than the breakneck speed at which you approached it.

Learn to love exercise.

Working out may be a national trend, but there are plenty of us who can't understand why folks get so hooked on grunting and panting and sweating. It's not fun; it's work! The doubters among us have likely never had pleasant experiences with exercise. They may have tried a workout or two but felt uncomfortable at it and never picked it up again.

You've heard the old folks saying, "You do what you want to do." That means you won't let anything get in the way of doing something you love. One of the surest ways of falling in love with exercise is to start slowly, to choose an activity that you enjoy, and to do it consistently.

Starting too quickly and with too high a goal can cause a momentum-sapping injury—or worse. A 1999 report from the American Medical Association indicated that sedentary folks who suddenly started vigorous exercise have a much greater risk of heart attack. Take it slow at first, then build up.

Think about what kinds of things you're already interested in—dancing, martial arts, biking, boxing—and choose an exercise based on that. Then give it a chance. When you don't exercise regularly, you deny yourself the chance to discover the rhythm of the movement. If you feel out of sync with the exercise, it's not much fun.

Surround yourself with like-minded people.

Have you noticed how difficult it can be to be with people who don't share your values? They want to light up; you're afraid of the secondhand smoke. You look forward to your afternoon date with the treadmill; they complain you spend too much time at the gym. You like your quiet time;

they're blasting the stereo. It's difficult to be in an environment that feels mismatched or even hostile to your needs. It's so much easier to be around like-minded people, people who support your weight-loss efforts and who may even be traveling a holistic-health journey similar to yours.

A synergy can develop between like-minded people, so that one person learns from another, they encourage and support each other, and they help each other find answers to the questions that they all encounter. This kind of communion brings tangible and measurable benefits as well as emotional ones: Scientists say people who exercise with buddies stick with their workout programs and lose significantly more weight than do folks who go at it solo.

Look for Divine guidance every day.

People of African descent are deeply spiritual people. Many, if not most of us, believe that our lives are guided and safeguarded by something infinitely larger than ourselves. This Divine influence has various names, but whether your sense of spirituality is grounded in Christianity, Islam, Buddhism, or simply an intuitive sense that everything in the universe unfolds according to a Divine plan, we gain strength from placing our faith and trust in that power force.

As you go about your new lifestyle, it can be tremendously comforting to remember that you're being guided by a greater power. Belief in this Divine presence makes your journey a little more certain and gives you the confidence that comes from knowing that you're being watched over and assisted every step of the way.

10 Keys to Healthy Weight Maintenance

You've heard it all before, but here's a quick refresher course from our nutrition expert Constance Brown-Riggs.

1. *Take a personal inventory.* Determine what changes need to be made in your body and your life. What is your motivation for making these changes. Do you want to lose ten pounds for a wedding? Do you have

diabetes and need to reduce your caloric intake to facilitate lowering your blood sugar levels? Are you losing weight for someone else?

2. *Set reasonable expectations.* Small, gradual changes usually work best. Drastic ones tend to be short-lived. You didn't put the weight on or develop poor eating habits overnight—and you aren't going to change them overnight.

   Set a goal range rather than a single specific weight. When outlining these goals, consider family weight patterns and history as well as your own previous weight history.

3. *Make sure your meals are nutritionally adequate.* Make legumes/beans, whole grains, fresh fruit, and vegetables a central part of your meal plan. These are low-fat, high-fiber foods that contain fewer calories, gram for gram, than foods high in fat. Proteins and carbohydrates have 4 calories per gram, while fat has 9 calories per gram.

4. *Make sure your meals are balanced.* Look at your plate. A third or less should be meat or protein and the other two-thirds to three-quarters should be grains and vegetables. Follow a food pyramid for daily serving recommendations.

5. *Slow down.* The satiety signal sends the brain a message after twenty minutes of eating: This body is full. Learning to eat more slowly can translate into eating less without feeling hungry. Put your fork down after each mouthful; and take time to chew your food well before swallowing. Only then should you pick up your fork for the next mouthful.

6. *Don't let your body feel deprived.* Eat a minimum of three meals a day. But even smaller, more frequent meals work because they help keep the metabolism revved up and hunger pangs down. Just don't eat frequent, small meals of doughnuts and coffee, pretzels and soda, pasta in alfredo sauce . . . you get the picture.

Don't skip meals, either. This can lead you to overeat at the next meal. Take relaxation breaks and try not to get too tired. If you don't have much energy, it's easy to yield to temptation.

7. *Become a label reader.* The nutrition label on the back of almost all foods can help you steer clear of high-calorie, high-fat foods. When you're looking at labels, look for foods with no more than 3 grams of total fat per 100 calories—and don't forget to look at the serving size.

8. *Drink plenty of water.* Sip eight glasses or more of water daily to help fill the stomach and to dilute metabolic wastes that are formed from the breakdown of fat. It also helps keep your skin clear and your digestive system running smoothly.

9. *Get active.* Participate in some form of regular physical activity above and beyond your regular daily movements. Expending enough energy—that is at least twenty to thirty minutes of vigorous exercise five to six days a week—is key to weight loss.

10. *Persevere and persist.* If at first you don't succeed, try, try again. Take it one meal at a time and put things in proper perspective. There are at least twenty-one meals in a week. If you overeat at one or even two of them, all is not lost. You can make up for it before the week is over.

   If you decide to have something fattening, make sure it's so good that it's worth it. Tell yourself that instead of nibbling on a couple of stale, store-bought cookies, you'll reserve the calories for one of your auntie's hot, homemade ones. Then savor and enjoy every bite.

   Don't beat yourself up over occasional indulgences, but if you find that your bad days outweigh your good days, consider getting help from a registered dietitian, doctor, or counselor.

Continuing the Journey

Now we've come to the end of the road. You've studied, you've worked hard, and in the words of Frankie Beverly, you've felt the "joy and pain, sunshine and rain" that come with unlearning old habits and incorporating new ones into your life. Now it's time for you to continue your healthy lifestyle on your own. Don't worry, we'll always be here to help you; you can study this book over and over again—and you can always log on to our website (www.healthquestmag.com) for healthy lifestyle tips and support. But for the most part, you'll have to stand on your own two feet.

This is your life; all the decisions are yours. Our Creator gave human beings free will and we have no choice but to use it. Now's the time to make your first set of choices.

Starting today, starting right now, are you going to choose to build upon the positive momentum you've created, or will you backslide into old habits again? Either way is fine, although each choice has its consequences. Of course, we hope you'll choose good habits and good health, especially now that you know the potentially disastrous health consequences that await folks who make unhealthy choices time and time again. Our community, our families, our children desperately need you alive and vibrant.

Still, lapsing back into old habits doesn't have to be a terminal or irreversible condition. Each day, each meal, each food choice, presents us with an opportunity to start over, to choose again and choose differently. You'll find that each day builds upon the momentum of the previous day and good choices gather momentum just as bad ones do. Over time, healthy living gets easier and easier; before you know it, it will be second nature. But in the beginning, changing your lifestyle can be very hard work. You're certain to slip up and have regrets. But God doesn't expect you to be perfect, so you shouldn't either. Just use your next choice to choose differently. We are human beings in the process of being human, and life is all about growing and changing. As the young folks say, *It's all good.*

Appendix 1

Nutritional Information

This section contains nutritional information for many common traditional and soul foods. Refer to it when you want to know how many calories and fat grams are in the foods you plan to eat. The data for the vegetables assumes they are boiled; unless otherwise indicated, the calorie count for meats assumes they have been baked, broiled, grilled, poached, roasted, or steamed. Use these numbers as approximate figures, depending on cooking method.

Another great planning tool is the U.S. Food Exchange System, which was developed to help people with diabetes control their carbohydrate and fat consumption. Though for diabetics, this system is useful for any person trying to plan a diet based on calorie control and limiting fats. *Exchange Lists for Meal Planning* can be ordered from the American Diabetes Association (800-232-3472) or the American Dietetic Association (800-366-1655).

Food	Serving Size	Calories	Fat Grams
Soups			
Bean	1 cup	173	5.9
Cream-of soups	1 cup	125	8
Split pea	1 cup	189	4.4
Tomato	1 cup	86	1.9
Vegetable beef, chicken, or other broth type	1 cup	25	1
Vegetables			
Baked potato flesh/skin	1 med.	88	0.2
Beets, sliced	1 cup	58	0.1
Broccoli	1 cup	25	0.5
Cabbage	1 cup	16	0.4
Collard greens	1 cup	57	0.3
Corn	1 cup	144	0.1
Dandelion	1 cup	24	0.6
Eggplant	1 cup	21	0.2
Hot chili peppers raw	½ cup	27	0.2
Kale	1 cup	33	0.5
Mustard greens	1 cup	14	0.4

Food	Serving Size	Calories	Fat Grams
Okra, raw	1 cup	38	0.3
Poke salad	1 cup	32	0.4
Rutabagas	1 cup	50	0.8
Spinach	1 cup	12	0.5
Squash, yellow	1 cup	26	0.6
String snap beans/beans	1 cup	34	0.2
Succotash	½ cup	145	0.8
Sweet potato, baked	1 small	136	0.1
Sweet potato, candied	1 piece	324	3
Tomatoes, raw	1 cup	37	0.3
Turnip greens	1 cup	14	0.3
Turnips, diced	1 cup	35	0.2

Fruits

Food	Serving Size	Calories	Fat Grams
Apple	1 med.	60	0
Cantaloupe	1 cup	60	0
Grapefruit	½ med.	24	0
Grapes	1 cup	101	
Honeydew	1 cup	60	0
Muscadine	17	60	1
Orange	1 med.	60	0
Peach	1 med.	60	0
Pear	1 med.	270	0
Plum	1 med.	60	0
Strawberries	¼ cup	27	0.7
Watermelon	1 cup	48	1

Grains/Starch

Food	Serving Size	Calories	Fat Grams
Biscuits	1	276	0
Cornbread	1 slice	188	4
Farina	½ cup	58	0.1
Grits, hominy	¾ cup	434	1
Macaroni	½ cup	194	0.5
Muffins, plain	1	168	4
Oatmeal	½ cup	149	1
Rice, brown	½ cup	343	2.8
Rice, white	½ cup	337	3.6

Meat

Food	Serving Size	Calories	Fat Grams
Beef liver, fried	1 oz.	40	5
Chicken liver	½ cup	147	4
Neckbone, fresh	3 oz.	225	12
Frog legs, steamed	4 legs	292	0

Food	Serving Size	Calories	Fat Grams
Gizzards, chicken	½ cup	139	3
Ham hock	2 oz.	62	13
Hog brains	1 oz.	112	3
Hog jowl	3 oz.	156	8
Kidney, pork	2 ½ oz.	105	3
Loin roast lean pork	3 oz.	131	12
Opossum	3 oz.	165	9
Oxtail	3 oz.	216	11
Pig ears	3 oz.	165	9
Pig feet	1 foot	31	9
Pig tails (⅓ tail)	1 oz.	113	10
Pork chop, lean	2 oz.	87	15
Sausage, link, pork	2	236	8
Sousemeat/headcheese, pork	2 oz.	120	9
Spareribs	2 oz.	100	17
Squirrel, roasted	3 oz.	102	4
Sweetbreads, pork	1 oz.	47	2
Tongue, pork	3 oz.	225	16
Tripe, pork	2 oz.	79	2
Turtle	3 oz.	120	3
Venison	3 oz.	153	3
Vienna sausage, pork	2 small	89	8
Wild rabbit, stewed	3 oz.	97	3

Fish

Food	Serving Size	Calories	Fat Grams
Catfish, fried	3 oz.	80	11
Crab cake	2 oz.	88	4
Croaker, fried	3 oz.	88	11
Flounder	3 oz.	57	1
Mullet, cooked dry	3 oz.	99	4
Oysters, moist heat	3 oz.	57	4
Perch, fried	3 oz.	77	7
Red snapper, cooked dry	3 oz.	85	2
Sardines, canned/oil	2 oz.	117	6
Shrimp, moist heat	3 oz.	84	1
Trout	3 oz.	125	10
Whiting, cooked dry	3 oz.	76	1
Sole	3 oz.	100	1
Salmon	3 oz.	175	11

Poultry

Food	Serving Size	Calories	Fat Grams
Chicken wing, roasted	3 oz.	247	17
Chicken drumstick, meat and skin	3 oz.	184	10

Food	Serving Size	Calories	Fat Grams
Chicken breast, meat only	3 oz.	140	3
Chicken thigh, meat only	3 oz.	178	9
Turkey breast, light meat	3 oz.	120	.9
Turkey drumstick	3 oz.	140	4

Beef

Porterhouse steak, choice broiled	3 oz.	185	9
T-Bone steak, broiled	3 oz.	182	9
Ground beef, regular fat, pan fried	3 oz.	243	16
Ground beef, extra lean, grilled	3 oz.	233	13

Combination Foods

Casseroles, chili with beans	1 cup	300	4
Chili with beans	1 cup	300	4
Chow mein (beef, chicken, or pork)	2 cups	525	10
Fried rice	1 cup	370	12
Pasta (lasagna, macaroni with cheese, spaghetti with meatballs)	1 cup	300	22
Pot pies	1	395	31

Fast Foods

Baked potato, super stuffed	1	610	22
Bean burrito	1	370	12
Chicken breast and wing, breaded, deep fried	1	540	
Chicken nuggets,	6 pieces	300	18
Chicken sandwich, breaded, deep fried	1	500	21
Fish sandwich	1	360	17
French fries, thin	20–25	250	13
Hamburger, deluxe	¼ pound	700	45
Hot dog on a bun	1	225	12
Ice cream, soft serve (medium)	1 cone	205	7
Pizza, deluxe	2 slices	618	28
Submarine sandwich	6 inch	420	21
Taco salad with chips	1	680	25

Dairy Products

Cheese, full fat	1 oz.	114	9
Cheese, low fat	1 oz.	66	3
Cottage cheese, full fat	½ cup	79	4.7
Cottage cheese, low fat	½ cup	72	1.2
Milk, full fat	1 cup	150	8
Milk, 2% fat	1 cup	130	5

Food	Serving Size	Calories	Fat Grams
Milk, 1% fat	1 cup	110	5
Milk, skim	1 cup	80	0
Yogurt, full fat	½ cup	79	3
Yogurt, low fat	½ cup	56	0.8

Fats and Oils

Butter	1 tbsp.	100	11
Cooking Oil	1 tbsp.	124	14
Lard	1 tbsp.	114	13
Margarine	1 tbsp.	101	11

Condiments

Horseradish sauce	1 tbsp.	6	0
Margarine	1 tbsp.	101	11
Mayonnaise, regular	1 tbsp.	100	11
Mayonnaise, low fat	1 tbsp.	43	4.2
Mustard	1 tsp.	5	0
Salad dressing, regular	1 tbsp.	70	9
Salad dressing, low fat	1 tbsp.	30–50	3–5
Seafood cocktail sauce	1 tbsp.	20	0

Desserts

Angel food, chocolate, unfrosted	1 slice	228	13
Cookies, chocolate chip	2 cookies	100	4.5
Ice cream, vanilla	¾ cup	194	9.8
Pies and Cobblers			
—Apple	⅛ pie	300	12
—Coconut Custard	⅛ pie	263	13
—Lemon Meringue	⅛ pie	338	13
—Mincemeat	⅛ pie	413	24
—Peach	⅛ pie	300	13
—Pecan	⅛ pie	413	24
—Sweet Potato	⅛ pie	225	13

Snacks

Peanuts	1 oz.	220	20
Popcorn	1 oz.	150	10
Potato chips	1 oz.	150	10
Tortilla chips	1 oz.	150	8

Beverages

Water or seltzer	20 oz.	0	
Diet soda	20 oz.	5	

Food	Serving Size	Calories	Fat Grams
Coffee, with one liquid creamer	8 oz.	30	
Tea, with two packets sugar	8 oz.	50	
Beer, light	12 oz.	100	
Beer, regular	12 oz.	150	
Starbucks cappuccino, short	8 oz.	100	
Apple or orange juice	8 oz.	110	
Iced tea, sweetened	16 oz.	120	
Gatorade	20 oz.	130	
Mimosa	8 oz.	150	
Wine, white	8 oz.	160	
Gin and tonic	7.5 oz	170	
Soda (cola, lemon-lime, etc.)	20 oz.	250	
Soda (cola, lemon-lime, etc.)	32 oz.	300	
Soda (cola, lemon-lime, etc.)	64 oz.	600	

Appendix 2

HealthQuest Two-Week Menu Plan

Week I

Day 1

Breakfast
½ cup cooked oatmeal
2 tablespoon raisins
1 cup light soy milk
1 teaspoon margarine
Calorie-free beverage

Lunch
2 slices low-calorie whole-wheat
 bread
2 ounces lean fresh ham
1 cup raw carrot sticks
1 small apple
1 teaspoon russian dressing
Calorie-free beverage

Dinner
2 ounces JAMAICAN JERK
 CHICKEN
1 cup CARIBBEAN RICE
 AND PEAS
2 cups tossed salad
2 tablespoons vinaigrette salad
 dressing
1 small orange
Calorie-free beverage

Snack
1 cup soy vanilla yogurt
Calorie-free beverage

Day 2

Breakfast
½ multigrain bagel
½ grapefruit
1 soy veggie slice
Calorie-free beverage

Lunch
2 slices low-calorie whole-wheat
 bread
2 ounces roast turkey breast
Lettuce leaves
½ cup THREE-BEAN SALAD
1 teaspoon mayonnaise
Calorie-free beverage

Dinner
1 cup cooked garlic and pasta
2 ounces (90%) fat-free ground beef
½ cup tomato sauce
2 cups escarole
1 square MAMA-NEVER-
 MADE-IT-LIKE-THAT PEACH
 COBBLER

Snack

1/2 cup tapioca pudding

Calorie-free beverage

Day 3

Breakfast

3/4 cup Cheerios

1/2 banana

1/2 cup skim milk

Calorie-free beverage

Lunch

2 ounces water-packed tuna

1 cup arugula, romaine, and
   chicory salad

1 cup asparagus spears

1 medium kiwi fruit

1 tablespoon Italian dressing

Calorie-free beverage

Dinner

1 GREAT BIG BISCUIT

1/2 cup CLASSIC MACARONI AND
   CHEESE

1/2 TANTALIZING, CRISPY OVEN-
   FRIED CHICKEN

1/2 cup French-style green beans

1 teaspoon margarine

Calorie-free beverage

Snack

3 ginger snap cookies

1 cup herbal tea

Day 4

Breakfast

2 small buttermilk pancakes

1 ounce maple syrup

1/2 cup chilled orange juice

1 teaspoon margarine

Calorie-free beverage

Lunch

1 cup STICK-TO-YOUR-RIBS
   BLACK BEAN SOUP

1 1/2 cups tossed salad greens

1 medium tomato

2 tablespoons low-calorie French
   salad dressing

1 small pear

Calorie-free beverage

Dinner

1/3 cup fluffy brown rice

2 ounces SCRUMPTIOUS MEAT
   LOAF

1 cup steamed broccoli

1 cup cantaloupe cubes

1 teaspoon margarine

Calorie-free beverage

Snack

1 slice SENSATIONAL SWEET
   POTATO PIE

1 1/2 cup fat-free vanilla ice cream

Day 5

Breakfast

1 slice rye toast
1 soft-boiled egg
1 tablespoon strawberry
    spreadable fruit
1 teaspoon margarine
Calorie-free beverage

Lunch

1 slice pizza (1/8 of a pie)
1 cup sesame spinach salad
2 small plums
1 teaspoon sesame oil
Calorie-free beverage

Dinner

1 slice SPICY CORN PONE
2 ounces CRISY OVEN-FRIED
    FISH with lemon
1/2 cup FINGER-LICKING
    SMOTHERED GREENS
1 cup mixed vegetable salad
1 tablespoon French dressing
Calorie-free beverage

Snack

1 cup strawberry smoothie with
1 cup light soy milk
1 1/4 cups strawberries

Day 6

Breakfast

1/2 cup cooked Wheatina
3 stewed prunes
1 cup skim milk
Calorie-free beverage

Lunch

1/3 cup fluffy brown rice
1/2 cup BEST-EVER RED BEAN
    CHILI
Crisp lettuce wedge
1 teaspoon bacon bits
17 grapes
1 tablespoon reduced-fat blue
    cheese dressing
Calorie-free beverage

Dinner

1 light hamburger bun
2 ounces BEST-EVER BURGER
    with
1 teaspoon ketchup
1 cup green salad with
FRUITED VINEGAR salad
    dressing
1/2 cup unsweetened canned
    peaches
Calorie-free beverage

Snack

1 (3") whole-wheat pita
1 1/2 teaspoons peanut butter
1 cup skim milk

Day 7

Breakfast

1 sliced fresh peach
2 slices French toast made with
    low-calorie bread
1 ounce maple syrup
1 teaspoon margarine
Calorie-free beverage

Lunch

8 ounces BEST-EVER RED
  BEAN CHILI

½ ounce shredded cheese

1 cup green salad with

1 tablespoon ranch dressing

½ cup canned unsweetened apricots

Calorie-free beverage

Dinner

2 ounces SCRUMPTIOUS
  MEAT LOAF

⅓ cup long-grain rice

1 cup assorted frozen melon balls

Calorie-free beverage

Snack

1 slice IRRESISTIBLE
  GINGERBREAD

Calorie-free beverage

Week 2

Day 1

Breakfast

½ cup cooked grits

¾ cup carrot juice

2 egg-white omelet

1 ounce low-fat cheese

1 slice whole-wheat toast

1 teaspoon margarine

Calorie-free beverage

Lunch

1 (3") whole-wheat pita

2 ounces lamb kabob

Lettuce and tomato

17 grapes

1 ounce cucumber dill sauce

Calorie-free beverage

Dinner

1 small baked potato (3 ounces)

2 ounces broiled chicken
  (remove all skin)

1 cup broccoli

½ cup mandarin orange sections
  in light syrup

1 teaspoon margarine

Calorie-free beverage

Snack

1 cup light soy milk

3 ginger snap cookies

Day 2

Breakfast

1 light whole-grain English muffin

⅛ honeydew

1 teaspoon margarine

Calorie-free beverage

Lunch

1 slice multigrain bread

½ cup water-packed tuna on a bed
  of romaine lettuce

2 small clementines

1 teaspoon mayonnaise

Calorie-free beverage

Dinner

1 cup basmati rice

2 ounces FINGER-LICKING
  CURRIED CHICKEN

1 cup French-style green beans
½ cup fruit cocktail in light syrup
Calorie-free beverage

Snack
½ cup low-fat rice pudding
1 cup herbal tea

Day 3

Breakfast
½ cup raisin bran cereal
½ banana
½ cup light soy milk
Calorie-free beverage

Lunch
1 light hamburger bun
2 ounces veggie burger
1 large tomato
1 cup raspberries
1 teaspoon honey mustard
Calorie-free beverage

Dinner
½ cup SOULFUL SPANISH RICE
2 ounces lean pork loin
1 cup steamed cabbage
1 ¼ cups fresh strawberries
Calorie-free beverage

Snack
3 graham crackers
Calorie-free beverage

Day 4

Breakfast
1 ½ cups puffed wheat
1 small orange
½ cup skim milk
Calorie-free beverage

Lunch
1 hard deli roll (2 ounces)
2 ounces lean roast beef
2 lettuce leaves
1 cup CARROT-RAISIN SALAD
Calorie-free beverage

Dinner
1 ¼ cups VITAL VEGETABLE
STEW
1 cup green salad
2 tablespoons fat-free dressing
1 dinner roll
Calorie-free beverage

Snack
1 cup SUMMER BREEZES
SMOOTHIE

Day 5

Breakfast
1 low-fat corn muffin
2 scrambled egg whites
1 tablespoon spreadable fruit
1 teaspoon margarine
Calorie-free beverage

Lunch

1 slice pizza (⅛ of a pie)

Small green salad with lettuce and
    tomatoes

2 small plums

1 teaspoon salad dressing

Calorie-free beverage

Dinner

1 cup FIERY OVEN FRENCH
    FRIES

2 ounces LIP-SMACKING ZESTY
    FISH

1 cup mixed vegetables

1 nectarine

Calorie-free beverage

Snack

1 cup apple soy yogurt

Day 6

Breakfast

½ cup cooked oatmeal

½ grapefruit

½ cup skim milk

Calorie-free beverage

Lunch

1 cup SCRUMPTIOUS RED
    BEANS AND RICE

1 cup arugula, romaine, and chicory
    salad

17 grapes

1 tablespoon French dressing

Calorie-free beverage

Dinner

1 small baked potato

3 ounces SPICY SOUTHERN
    BARBECUED CHICKEN

1 cup cooked green beans

½ cup unsweetened canned peaches

1 teaspoon margarine

Calorie-free beverage

Snack

½ cup baked caramel custard

Day 7

Breakfast

2 (4") buttermilk pancakes

1 ounce maple syrup

¾ cup blueberries

1 teaspoon margarine

Calorie-free beverage

Lunch

½ cup QUICK JUMPING
    JAMBALAYA

1 cup tossed salad

1 small fresh apple

Calorie-free beverage

Dinner

1 slice GOOD-FOR-YOU
    CORNBREAD

⅓ cup steamed rice

4 ounces COME-'N-GET-IT
    FARMLAND RIBS

1 cup fresh okra

Calorie-free beverage

Snack

3 chocolate wafers

1 cup herbal tea

Appendix 3

HealthQuest Recipes*

Spicy Corn Pone

Good-for-You Cornbread

Great Big Biscuits

Fiery Oven French Fries

Savory Potato Salad

Three-Bean Salad

Carrot-Raisin Salad

Best-Ever Red Bean Chili

Finger-Licking Smothered Greens

Scrumptious Red Beans and Rice

Vital Vegetable Stew

Caribbean Rice and Peas

Stick-to-Your-Ribs Black Bean Soup

Soulful Spanish Rice

Jamaican-Style Jerk Chicken

Finger-Licking Curried Chicken

Tantalizing Crispy Oven-Fried Chicken

Classic Macaroni and Cheese

Quick Jumping Jambalaya

Shameless Chicken Gumbo

Spicy Southern Barbecued Chicken

Crispy Oven-Fried Fish

Lip-Smacking Zesty Fish

Scrumptious Meat Loaf

Come-'n-Get-It Farmland Ribs

Recipes by Goulda Downer, Ph.D., R.D., C.N.S., Metroplex Health and Nutrition Services, Inc.

Best-Ever Burger

Sensational Mock Sweet Potato Pie

Irresistible Gingerbread

Mama-Never-Made-It-Like-That Peach Cobbler

Summer Breezes Smoothie

Fruited Vinegar

 ## SPICY CORN PONE

2 cups yellow cornmeal

½ cup all-purpose flour

2 teaspoons baking powder, low sodium

4 ounces whole kernel corn, low sodium

½ cup chopped onion

1 egg, well beaten

2 cups water

1 tablespoon olive oil

1 small green chili pepper, chopped

1 small red chili pepper, chopped

⅛ teaspoon ground red pepper

⅛ teaspoon ground white pepper

2 tablespoons chopped yellow bell pepper

2 tablespoons chopped red bell pepper

2 tablespoons chopped green bell pepper

1. Preheat oven to 400 degrees Fahrenheit.
2. Combine all ingredients together in a large bowl.
3. Bake in nonstick 8-inch pan for 30 to 40 minutes or until a knife inserted in center comes out clean.
4. Cut into 6 squares.

SERVING SIZE: 1 SQUARE. MAKES 6 SERVINGS.

Calories 277 • Fat 5 g • Saturated Fat 1 g
Cholesterol 35 mg • Sodium 30 mg

GOOD-FOR-YOU CORNBREAD

1 cup yellow cornmeal

1 cup all-purpose flour

½ cup brown sugar

1 tablespoon baking powder, low sodium

¼ teaspoon salt

1 teaspoon cinnamon

1 teaspoon nutmeg

⅓ cup applesauce, unsweetened

1 cup buttermilk

1 tablespoon vanilla extract

2 egg whites

1. Preheat oven to 400 degrees Fahrenheit.
2. Stir cornmeal, flour, sugar, baking powder, salt, cinnamon, and nutmeg in a large bowl.
3. In another bowl, stir applesauce, buttermilk, vanilla, and egg whites together.
4. Add the applesauce mixture to the cornmeal mixture and stir until moistened.
5. Pour the batter into lightly greased 8-inch square pan.
6. Bake about 25 to 35 minutes until golden brown and a knife inserted in center comes out clean.
7. Cut into 12 squares.

SERVING SIZE: 1 SQUARE. MAKES 12 SERVINGS.

Calories   193

Fat   1 g

Saturated Fat   less than 1 g

Cholesterol   less than1 mg

Sodium   83 mg

GREAT BIG BISCUITS

2 cups all-purpose flour

1 cup whole-wheat flour

½ teaspoon cream of tartar

1 teaspoon baking powder, low sodium

⅛ teaspoon salt

3 tablespoons sugar

1 tablespoon soft tub margarine

1 cup evaporated skim milk

1 egg, well beaten

1. Preheat oven to 425 degrees Fahrenheit.
2. Combine all dry ingredients in a bowl.
3. Add margarine and crumble into dry mixture until it resembles coarse cornmeal.
4. Mix milk and beaten egg in separate dish. Add to flour crumble mixture.
5. Knead lightly on floured board.
6. Roll or shape by hand into 1-inch thickness and cut into 12 biscuits.
7. Place on nonstick baking trays.
8. Bake for 15 to 20 minutes.

SERVING SIZE: 1 BISCUIT. MAKES 12 SERVINGS.

Calories   243

Fat   2 g

Saturated Fat   less than 1g

Cholesterol   16 mg

Sodium   97 mg

FIERY OVEN FRENCH FRIES

4 large potatoes (about 2 pounds)
8 cups ice water
1 tablespoon garlic powder
1 teaspoon onion powder
½ teaspoon salt
1 tablespoon white pepper
¼ teaspoon allspice
1 teaspoon hot pepper flakes
2 tablespoons olive oil

1. Preheat oven to 475 degrees Fahrenheit.
2. Scrub potatoes and cut into long ½-inch-wide strips.
3. Place potato strips into ice water, cover, and chill for 1 hour or longer.
4. Remove potatoes and dry strips thoroughly.
5. Place garlic powder, onion powder, salt, white pepper, allspice, and hot pepper flakes in plastic bag.
6. Toss potatoes in pepper mixture.
7. Brush potatoes with olive oil.
8. Place potatoes in nonstick shallow baking pan.
9. Bake for 30 to 40 minutes or until golden brown. Turn fries occasionally to brown on all sides.

SERVING SIZE: 1 CUP. MAKES 4 SERVINGS.

Calories 325
Fat 7 g
Saturated Fat 1 g
Cholesterol 0
Sodium 25 mg

SAVORY POTATO SALAD

2 pounds potatoes, peeled

2 stalks celery, finely chopped

2 stalks scallion, finely chopped

¼ teaspoon finely chopped fresh garlic

1 small jalapeño pepper, finely chopped

1 medium red bell pepper, coarsely chopped

1 medium yellow bell pepper, coarsely chopped

1 medium green bell pepper, coarsely chopped

2 tablespoons finely chopped onion

3 tablespoons finely chopped fresh chives

2 teaspoons finely chopped fresh basil

1 tablespoon light cream

½ cup fat-free mayonnaise

1 teaspoon ground white pepper

1 teaspoon mustard

1 tablespoon granulated sugar

1. Cut potatoes into 2-inch squares.
2. Boil potatoes until tender but still firm.
3. Drain and cool potatoes then set aside.
4. Add vegetables to potatoes and toss.
5. Blend together cream, mayonnaise, white pepper, mustard, and sugar.
6. Pour dressing over potato mixture and stir gently to coat evenly.
7. Chill for at least 1 hour before serving.

SERVING SIZE: ½ CUP. MAKES 8 SERVINGS.

Calories   287

Fat   6 g

Saturated Fat   2 g

Cholesterol   8 mg

Sodium   134 mg

THREE-BEAN SALAD

1 can (15 ounces) chickpeas or cow peas, drained and rinsed

1 can (15 ounces) low-sodium kidney beans, drained and rinsed

1 can (15 ounces) black-eyed peas, drained and rinsed

2 stalks scallion, chopped

1 tablespoon chopped fresh garlic

1 tablespoon finely chopped leek

½ teaspoon chopped fresh cilantro (optional)

½ teaspoon finely chopped jalapeño pepper

½ cup coarsely chopped yellow bell pepper

½ cup coarsely chopped green bell pepper

½ cup coarsely chopped red bell pepper

1 tablespoon tomato paste, low sodium

½ teaspoon ground cumin

1 tablespoon vinegar

2 tablespoons olive oil

1. Drain the canned peas and beans then rinse under running cold water.
2. Add all the chopped vegetables to peas and bean mixture.
3. In a separate bowl, stir together tomato paste and remaining spices.
4. Pour over peas and beans mixture.
5. Chill for at least 1 hour before serving.

SERVING SIZE: 1 CUP. MAKES 8 SERVINGS.

Calories 285

Fat 3g

Saturated Fat less than 1 g

Cholesterol 0

Sodium 104 mg

CARROT-RAISIN SALAD

1 pound carrots, coarsely shredded

8 ounces crushed pineapple (drained)

½ cup seedless raisins

1 cup fat-free or nonfat plain or vanilla yogurt

¼ teaspoon orange extract

½ teaspoon vanilla extract

1. Combine carrots, pineapple, and raisins in a large bowl. Set aside.
2. Mix remaining ingredients together in a small bowl. Pour over carrot mixture and fold in.
3. Cover and chill for 1 to 2 hours.

SERVING SIZE: 1 CUP. MAKES 4 SERVINGS.

Calories   186

Fat   less than 1 g

Saturated Fat   less than 1 g

Cholesterol   1 mg

Sodium   95 mg

BEST-EVER RED BEAN CHILI

1 tablespoon olive oil

1 large onion, chopped

2 stalks fresh scallion, chopped

2 pounds ripe tomatoes, finely chopped

2 tablespoons finely chopped garlic

1 tablespoon finely chopped leeks

3 cups water

4 ounces lentils, uncooked

2 stalks fresh thyme

1 tablespoon finely chopped hot pepper

½ teaspoon chili powder

2 tablespoons brown sugar

1 tablespoon low-sodium soy sauce

1 can (15 ounces) red kidney beans, drained and rinsed

1 stalk celery, chopped

½ cup tomato paste, low sodium

1. Heat oil in large skillet and sauté onion and scallion over moderate flame until brown.
2. Add tomatoes, garlic, and leeks, and cook for 15 minutes.
3. Add water, lentils, thyme, pepper, chili powder, 1 tablespoon brown sugar, and soy sauce.
4. Cover and simmer for 1 hour or until lentils are cooked. Stir occasionally.
5. Rinse kidney beans and add along with celery, salt, tomato paste, and the rest of sugar to lentil mixture.
6. Continue cooking for 15 minutes. Add additional water if needed.

SERVING SIZE: ½ CUP. MAKES 6 SERVINGS.

Calories   221

Fat   3 g

Saturated Fat   less than 1 g

Cholesterol   less than 1 g

Sodium   71 mg

FINGER-LICKING SMOTHERED GREENS

4 cups water

¼ pound skinless smoked turkey

¼ teaspoon liquid smoke (optional)

1 hot pepper, finely chopped

¼ teaspoon ground cloves

2 cloves garlic, crushed

1 teaspoon dried thyme

1 stalk scallion, chopped

1 teaspoon dried dill

1 teaspoon ground ginger

¼ cup chopped onion

2 pounds greens (mustard, turnip, collard, kale, or mixture)

1. Place all ingredients except greens into large saucepan and bring to a boil.
2. Prepare greens by washing thoroughly and removing stems.
3. Tear or slice leaves into bite-size pieces.
4. Add greens to turkey stock. Cook 20 to 30 minutes or until well done.

SERVING SIZE: 1 CUP. MAKES 4 SERVINGS.

Calories 62

Fat 2 g

Saturated Fat less than 1 g

Cholesterol 0

Sodium 29 mg

SCRUMPTIOUS RED BEANS AND RICE

2 cans (15 ounces each) red kidney beans, rinsed and drained

4 cups water

¼ pound skinless smoked turkey, cut in 1-inch cubes

1 large onion, chopped

1 stalk scallion, chopped

1 teaspoon dried thyme

1 small hot pepper, chopped

2 stalks celery and leaves (about ½ cup), chopped

2 cloves garlic, chopped

1. Rinse beans and place 1 can in large skillet.
2. Puree the other can and set aside.
3. Add turkey and let simmer for 15 minutes.
4. Add remaining spices to pot.
5. Stir in pureed beans until thickened.

    Serve on top of hot rice. (Can also be served on pasta, a warm roll, or eaten alone.)

SERVING SIZE: ½ CUP (BEANS ONLY). MAKES 8 SERVINGS.

Calories   176

Fat   5 g

Saturated Fat   less than 1 g

Cholesterol   less than 1 mg

Sodium   104 mg

VITAL VEGETABLE STEW

2 pounds summer squash, cut in 1-inch squares

1 pound white potatoes, cut in 2-inch strips

1 can (15 ounces) sweet corn, rinsed and drained
   (or 2 ears fresh corn)

1 pound carrots (cut into chunky wedges, or sliced, julienned,
   and diced—to add variation to the shape)

2 teaspoons dried thyme

1 teaspoon minced hot pepper

2 cloves garlic, minced

1 stalk scallion, chopped

1 teaspoon ground allspice

½ small hot pepper, chopped

1 low-sodium vegetable bouillon cube

1 cup coarsely chopped onion

6 cups water

(Add other preferred vegetables, such as broccoli, cauliflower, etc.)

1. Combine all ingredients in a large pot.
2. Simmer for 20 minutes on medium flame or until cooked.
3. Remove 1 cup of squash and puree.
4. Return pureed mixture to pot and let cook for 10 minutes more.
5. Remove from flame and let sit for 10 minutes to allow stew to
   thicken.

SERVING SIZE: 1 ¼ CUPS. MAKES 6 SERVINGS.

Calories   158
Fat   3 g
Saturated Fat   less than 1 g
Cholesterol   0
Sodium   64 mg

CARIBBEAN RICE AND PEAS

1 can (15 ounces) red kidney beans, drained
  (or 2 cups dry kidney beans, soaked then cooked)
3 cups water
2 cloves garlic, crushed
1 stalk scallion, chopped
1 teaspoon dried thyme
1 teaspoon chopped hot pepper
1 tablespoon coconut cream (optional)
3 cups rice, uncooked

1. In a skillet, combine all ingredients except for uncooked rice and bring to a boil for 5 minutes.
2. Add rice, stirring once with a fork, and bring to a boil.
3. Cover pot tightly and reduce heat.
4. Let cook for 20 to 30 minutes or until all liquid is absorbed and rice is tender.
5. Add small amount of additional water, if necessary.

SERVING SIZE: ½ CUP. MAKES 8 SERVINGS.

Calories   309
Fat   1 g
Saturated Fat   1 g
Cholesterol   0
Sodium   11 mg

STICK-TO-YOUR-RIBS BLACK BEAN SOUP

1 pound black beans
6 cups water
1 tablespoon corn oil
1 large onion, chopped
½ pound white potatoes, diced
¼ pound skinless smoked turkey breast
1 sprig thyme, crushed
1 stalk leeks, chopped
1 teaspoon dried oregano
1 sprig scallion, chopped
1 teaspoon dried rosemary
3 bay leaves, whole
3 cloves garlic, minced
1 teaspoon ground cumin
1 teaspoon minced hot pepper
2 teaspoon brown sugar

1. Soak beans overnight in 6 cups of cold water then drain. (Optional: Use 1 can beans [15 ounces], rinsed and drained.)
2. Combine beans in 4 quarts of cold water and bring to boil.
3. Reduce heat and simmer for 1 ½ to 2 hours or until beans are cooked.
4. Over medium flame, heat oil in nonstick skillet and sauté onion until tender. Add to cooked beans.
5. Add potatoes and smoked turkey and let cook for 10 minutes.
6. Add remaining ingredients.
7. Continue to cook over low flame, stirring occasionally.
8. Allow potatoes to mash out and thicken soup.

SERVING SIZE: 1 CUP. MAKES 6 SERVINGS.

**Calories 223 • Fat 5 g • Saturated Fat less than 1 g
Cholesterol 0 • Sodium 16 mg**

SOULFUL SPANISH RICE

1 medium onion, chopped

1 small green pepper, diced

1 tablespoon corn oil

2 pounds tomatoes, ripe red

½ pound carrots, diced

1 cup whole kernel corn, fresh or frozen, drained

1 teaspoon crushed hot pepper

1 tablespoon onion powder

1 tablespoon garlic powder

1 tablespoon dried thyme

⅛ teaspoon salt

3 cups cooked rice

1. Sauté onion and green pepper in oil until soft.
2. Stir in all other ingredients except rice.
3. Let stand for 1 minute, then add rice.
4. Cook on low flame a in tightly covered pot for 20 to 25 minutes.

SERVING SIZE: ½ CUP. MAKES 6 SERVINGS.

Calories   189

Fat   3 g

Saturated Fat   less than 1 g

Cholesterol   0

Sodium   73 mg

JAMAICAN-STYLE JERK CHICKEN

2 pounds chicken pieces, skinless (breast or drumstick)

3 tablespoons ground cloves

3 tablespoons garlic powder

3 tablespoons onion powder

3 tablespoons ground allspice

3 tablespoons ground black pepper

3 tablespoons chopped hot pepper

3 tablespoons dried oregano

3 tablespoons dried thyme

3 cloves garlic, finely chopped

1 cup pureed or finely chopped onion

1 teaspoon ground cinnamon

¼ cup vinegar

¼ cup brown sugar

1. Preheat oven to 375 degrees Fahrenheit.
2. Clean chicken and set aside.
3. Combine remaining ingredients in large bowl and rub well over chicken.
4. Marinate in the refrigerator for 6 or more hours.
5. Barbecue chicken over medium flame, or evenly space chicken on nonstick or lightly greased baking pan.
6. Bake for 40 to 60 minutes or until well done. Serve hot or cold.

SERVING SIZE: ½ BREAST OR 2 SMALL DRUMSTICKS.
   MAKES 6 SERVINGS.

Calories   301
Fat   6 g
Saturated Fat   2 g
Cholesterol   103 mg
Sodium   127 mg

FINGER-LICKING CURRIED CHICKEN

2 pounds chicken pieces, skinless (breast or drumstick)

2 to 4 tablespoons curry powder

1 teaspoon dried thyme

1 stalk scallion, chopped

1 tablespoon chopped hot pepper

1 teaspoon ground black pepper

8 cloves garlic, crushed

1 tablespoon grated fresh ginger

1 large onion, chopped

1 teaspoon salt

1 tablespoon olive oil

1 cup water

1 medium white potato, diced

1. Remove skin and trim away any visible fat from the chicken.
2. Season with curry powder, thyme, scallion, hot pepper, black pepper, garlic, ginger, onion, and salt.
3. Marinate for at least 2 hours in the refrigerator.
4. Heat oil in skillet over medium flame.
5. Add chicken and sauté. Save onion for later.
6. Add water and allow chicken to cook over medium flame for 30 minutes.
7. Add diced potato and small amount of additional water if needed.
8. Let cook for an additional 30 minutes.
9. Add onion and cook 15 minutes more or until meat is tender.

SERVING SIZE: ½ BREAST OR 2 SMALL DRUMSTICKS.

MAKES 6 SERVINGS.

Calories   272

Fat   6 g

Saturated Fat   2 g

Cholesterol   103 mg

Sodium   102 mg

TANTALIZING CRISPY OVEN-FRIED CHICKEN

1 teaspoon poultry seasoning

½ cup skim milk or buttermilk

1 cup cornflakes, crumbled

3 tablespoons onion powder

3 tablespoons garlic powder

2 tablespoons black pepper

1 teaspoon cayenne pepper

2 teaspoons ground ginger

1 teaspoon ground allspice

2 pounds chicken pieces, skinless (breast or drumstick)

1. Preheat oven to 375 degree Fahrenheit.
2. Add ½ teaspoon of poultry seasoning to milk.
3. Combine cornflakes with all other dry ingredients and place into a plastic bag.
4. Remove all skin or visible pieces of fat from chicken. Wash and pat dry.
5. Dip chicken into milk, shake to remove excess, then quickly shake in the seasoning bag to coat.
6. Let stand briefly until coating sticks to chicken.
7. Evenly space chicken on nonstick or lightly greased baking pan.
8. Bake 40 to 60 minutes until well done. Crumbs will form a crispy "skin." (Do not turn chicken during baking.)

SERVING SIZE: ½ BREAST OR 2 SMALL DRUMSTICKS.

MAKES 6 SERVINGS.

Calories   351

Fat   10 g

Saturated Fat   3 g

Cholesterol   128 mg

Sodium   164 mg

CLASSIC MACARONI AND CHEESE

2 cups macaroni
Nonstick spray
$\frac{1}{2}$ cup chopped onions
1 $\frac{1}{2}$ cups evaporated skim milk
1 tablespoon cornstarch
1 tablespoon garlic powder
1 tablespoon onion powder
1 teaspoon white pepper
10 ounces finely shredded, low-fat, low-sodium sharp
   Cheddar cheese

1. Cook macaroni according to directions. Drain and set aside.
2. Preheat oven to 350 degrees Fahrenheit.
3. Spray casserole dish with nonstick spray.
4. Lightly spray saucepan with nonstick spray.
5. Add onions to saucepan and sauté for about 3 minutes.
6. In another bowl, mix skim milk and cornstarch until smooth.
7. Pour this into onion mixture.
8. Add in garlic powder, onion powder, and white pepper, and stir briskly.
9. Cook and stir constantly over medium heat until thick and bubbly.
10. Remove pot from heat. Slowly stir in cheese until melted.
11. Stir the macaroni into the cheese sauce. Transfer mixture into the prepared casserole dish.
12. Bake for 25 minutes or until bubbly. Let stand and cool for 10 minutes before serving.

SERVING SIZE: $\frac{1}{2}$ CUP. MAKES 6 SERVINGS.

Calories   263
Fat   9 g
Saturated Fat   5 g
Cholesterol   36 mg
Sodium   302 mg

QUICK JUMPING JAMBALAYA

¼ pound skinless smoked turkey breast

1 tablespoon corn oil

¼ pound shrimp, uncooked

2 ½ cups water

1 pound tomatoes, red ripe, chopped

1 medium onion, chopped

2 cloves garlic, chopped

1 stalk leek, chopped

1 stalk scallion, chopped

1 sprig thyme, chopped

1 teaspoon minced hot pepper

1 teaspoon ground allspice

2 cups uncooked rice

1 medium red bell pepper, diced

1 medium green bell pepper, diced

1. Cut turkey into 1-inch cubes.
2. Brown turkey in oil in skillet over medium heat.
3. Add all remaining ingredients to skillet, except for rice and bell peppers. Stir occasionally and allow to boil.
4. Add rice, reduce heat, and cover pot tightly.
5. Let cook for 25 to 35 minutes.
6. Add bell peppers and continue cooking for 5 to 10 minutes more or until done.

SERVING SIZE: 1 CUP. MAKES 6 SERVINGS.

Calories 340

Fat 4 g

Saturated Fat 1 g

Cholesterol 45 mg

Sodium 60 mg

SHAMELESS CHICKEN GUMBO

Nonstick vegetable oil spray
¼ cup all-purpose flour
3 cups water or defatted chicken broth
1 ½ pounds skinless chicken breast
½ pound white potatoes, cubed
1 cup chopped onions
½ pound carrots, coarsely chopped
¼ cup chopped celery
6 cloves garlic, finely minced
2 stalks scallion, chopped
1 bay leaf, whole
1 teaspoon dried thyme
½ teaspoon ground black pepper
2 teaspoons hot pepper (such as jalapeño)
½ pound fresh okra

1. Lightly coat skillet with nonstick vegetable oil spray.
2. Heat skillet over medium heat.
3. Stir in flour until it darkens.
4. Slowly stir in the broth.
5. Add all ingredients except okra. Bring to a boil, then reduce heat and let simmer for 20 to 30 minutes.
6. Add okra and let cook for 15 to 20 minutes more.
7. Serve hot, alone or over warm rice.

SERVING SIZE: ¾ CUP. MAKES 6 SERVINGS.

Calories   340
Fat   11 g
Saturated Fat   3 g
Cholesterol   96 mg
Sodium   113 mg

SPICY SOUTHERN BARBECUED CHICKEN

½ cup vinegar

½ cup water

6 ounces low-sodium tomato paste

2 tablespoons brown sugar

1 teaspoon ground black pepper

1 tablespoon hot pepper flakes

½ teaspoon poultry seasoning

2 tablespoons onion powder

2 tablespoons garlic powder

2 tablespoons dried thyme

2 tablespoons grated fresh ginger

1 ½ pounds chicken pieces, skinless (breast or drumstick)

1. Preheat oven to 350 degrees Fahrenheit.
2. Combine all ingredients in saucepan, except for chicken.
3. Simmer for 15 minutes.
4. Remove all skin from chicken. Wash and pat dry.
5. Place chicken in large baking pan.
6. Brush chicken with ¼ of sauce mixture.
7. Cover with foil and bake on top rack of the oven for 20 minutes.
8. Turn chicken and pour on remaining sauce.
9. Bake uncovered for 20 to 30 minutes until chicken turns golden brown.

SERVING SIZE: ½ BREAST OR 2 SMALL DRUMSTICKS.

MAKES 6 SERVINGS.

Calories   293

Fat   9 g

Saturated Fat   3 g

Cholesterol   96 mg

Sodium   116 mg

CRISPY OVEN-FRIED FISH

2 pounds fish fillets (whiting, kingfish, sole)
1 tablespoon vinegar or lime juice
¼ teaspoon salt
2 tablespoons ground black pepper
½ cup skim milk or buttermilk
2 tablespoons onion powder
2 tablespoons garlic powder
½ cup cornflakes, crumbled

1. Preheat oven to 500 degree Fahrenheit.
2. Wipe fillet with vinegar or lime juice and pat dry.
3. Add salt and black pepper to milk.
4. Combine all other dry ingredients with cornflake crumbs and place onto a plate.
5. Let fillet sit in milk briefly. Remove and arrange on lightly oiled shallow baking dish.
6. Brush cornflake crumb mixture onto fillet.
7. Let stand briefly until coating sticks to fish.
8. Bake 10 to 15 minutes on middle oven rack; do not turn or baste.

SERVING SIZE: 4 OUNCES. MAKES 6 SERVINGS.

Calories   125
Fat   2 g
Saturated Fat   less than 1 g
Cholesterol   76 mg
Sodium   102 mg

LIP-SMACKING ZESTY FISH

¼ cup all-purpose flour

2 tablespoons ground black pepper

¼ teaspoon salt

2 tablespoons garlic powder

2 tablespoons onion powder

1 pound fish (king, snapper, catfish, or any large fish)

3 tablespoons lime or lemon juice

2 tablespoons corn oil

½ cup malt vinegar

1 tablespoon whole allspice berries

1 large onion, sliced (about 1 cup)

1 medium carrot, cut in strips (about ¼ pound)

1 whole bay leaf

1 medium yellow bell pepper, cut into circles

1 medium red bell pepper, cut into circles

1 whole jalapeño pepper, sliced (about 2 tablespoons)

1. Preheat oven to 500 degrees Fahrenheit.
2. Combine flour, black pepper, salt, garlic powder, and onion powder in a plastic bag.
3. Wipe fillet with lime or lemon juice. Do not pat dry.
4. Shake fish in plastic bag with flour mixture until coated.
5. Dust off excess flour mixture.
6. Let stand briefly until coating sticks to fish.
7. Arrange in nonstick or lightly greased shallow baking dish.
8. Bake 10 to 15 minutes on middle oven rack; do not turn or baste.
9. Remove fish from pan and place in glass dish to cool.
10. Combine oil, vinegar, allspice, onion, carrot, bay leaf, bell peppers, and hot pepper in skillet and cook over medium heat.
11. Remove from heat as soon as oil-vinegar mixture comes to boil.
12. Pour hot mixture over fish and cover tightly.

13. Let marinate for 15 to 30 minutes before serving. (The longer it sits, the better it tastes.) May be served cold, hot, or at room temperature. Spoon marinade and spices over fish when you serve.

SERVING SIZE: 4 OUNCES. MAKES 4 SERVINGS.

Calories 217 • Fat 4 g • Saturated Fat 1 g
Cholesterol 53 mg • Sodium 154 mg

SCRUMPTIOUS MEAT LOAF

1 pound extra-lean ground beef
1 can (6 ounces) low-sodium tomato paste
¼ cup chopped onion
1 teaspoon low-sodium mustard
½ teaspoon ground black pepper
½ teaspoon chopped jalapeño pepper
2 cloves garlic, chopped
2 stalks scallion, chopped
½ teaspoon ground ginger
¼ teaspoon ground nutmeg
1 teaspoon grated orange peel
1 teaspoon dried thyme
¼ cup bread crumbs, finely grated

1. Preheat oven to 450 degrees Fahrenheit.
2. Mix all ingredients together.
3. Place in a 1-pound loaf tin and bake for 60 minutes.
4. Drain liquid, raise oven temperature to broil, then broil for 20 minutes or until golden brown.

SERVING SIZE: 2-INCH-THICK SLICE. MAKES 6 SERVINGS.

Calories 240 • Fat 10 g • Saturated Fat 4 g
Cholesterol 47 mg • Sodium 127 mg

COME-'N-GET-IT FARMLAND RIBS

1 pound lean beef ribs, all fat trimmed off

3 tablespoons garlic powder

1 tablespoon ground black pepper

2 tablespoons onion powder

1/4 teaspoon salt

1 cup chopped onion

2 cloves garlic, minced

1/2 cup low-sodium tomato paste

1 cup water

4 tablespoons brown sugar

1/4 cup vinegar

1 tablespoon low-sodium mustard

1/4 teaspoon celery seed

1 teaspoon cayenne pepper

1 tablespoon grated orange peel

1. Rub ribs with garlic powder, black pepper, onion powder, and salt.
2. Cook ribs in microwave for 20 to 30 minutes.
3. Combine remaining ingredients in saucepan and simmer, uncovered, for 10 minutes, stirring occasionally.
4. Put ribs on grill over slow coal. Turn every 15 minutes for 45 to 60 minutes.
5. Brush with sauce until ribs are well coated.

SERVING SIZE: 4 OUNCES. MAKES 4 SERVINGS.

Calories 384
Fat 10 g
Saturated Fat 3 g
Cholesterol 163 mg
Sodium 146 mg

BEST-EVER BURGER

¼ cup regular beer

2 tablespoons fat-free ranch dressing

⅓ cup fine bread crumbs

¼ cup finely chopped onion

3 tablespoons garlic powder

2 tablespoons onion powder

1 teaspoon dried thyme

1 teaspoon chopped hot pepper

1 pound extra-lean ground beef

1. Combine beer and ranch dressing and set aside.
2. Combine all other ingredients in a bowl.
3. Add ground beef and half the beer-dressing mixture to the dry ingredients, and mix all together well.
4. Form into 8 patties (approximately ¾ inch thick).
5. Grill over medium heat for about 10 to 15 minutes until done.
6. Turn occasionally and baste with remaining beer-dressing mixture.

SERVING SIZE: 1 PATTY. MAKES 8 SERVINGS.

Calories   184
Fat   10 g
Saturated Fat   4 g
Cholesterol   38 mg
Sodium   135 mg

SENSATIONAL MOCK SWEET POTATO PIE

2 tablespoons all-purpose flour

3 cups cooked and pureed sweet potatoes (or yams)

1 egg, well beaten

½ cup evaporated skim milk

½ cup brown sugar

1 teaspoon ground nutmeg

1 teaspoon ground cinnamon

1 tablespoon vanilla extract

1 teaspoon ground ginger

1 tablespoon lemon juice

1. Preheat oven to 425 degrees Fahrenheit.
2. Sift flour over sweet potato in large bowl and mix.
3. Add all other ingredients and mix thoroughly.
4. Pour into lightly greased 12-inch pie dish.
5. Bake for 15 to 20 minutes, then reduce oven temperature to 350 degrees.
6. Bake until pie is golden brown or until knife inserted into the center comes out clean.
7. Let cool for 20 to 30 minutes. Cut into 8 equal slices.

SERVING SIZE: 1 SLICE. MAKES 8 SERVINGS.

Calories 196

Fat 1 g

Saturated Fat less than 1 g

Cholesterol 36 mg

Sodium 46 mg

IRRESISTIBLE GINGERBREAD

1 cup dark molasses

½ cup firmly packed brown sugar

¼ cup olive oil

2 tablespoons freshly grated ginger

1 teaspoon ground cinnamon

1 teaspoon ground nutmeg

2 tablespoons vanilla extract

½ teaspoon ground cloves

1 cup boiling water

2 ½ cups all-purpose flour, sifted

1 teaspoon low-sodium baking powder

1 teaspoon baking soda

2 tablespoons hot water

1. Preheat oven to 350 degrees Fahrenheit.
2. Blend molasses, brown sugar, oil, ginger, cinnamon, nutmeg, vanilla, and cloves together.
3. Stir in the boiling water.
4. Mix in flour and baking powder and set aside.
5. Dissolve baking soda in the 2 tablespoons of hot water.
6. Pour baking soda mixture into flour mixture and mix well.
7. Bake in nonstick 8-inch pan for 30 minutes or until knife inserted in center comes out clean.
8. Cut into 2-inch squares.

SERVING SIZE: 1 SQUARE. MAKES 12 SERVINGS.

Calories   231

Fat   5 g

Saturated Fat   1 g

Cholesterol   0

Sodium   98 mg

MAMA-NEVER-MADE-IT-LIKE-THAT PEACH COBBLER

$^1/_2$ cup granulated sugar

1 teaspoon ground cinnamon

1 tablespoon vanilla extract

2 tablespoons cornstarch

$^1/_4$ cup pineapple juice

8 ounces peach nectar

2 $^1/_2$ pounds peaches, canned in water, drained

1 tablespoon soft tub margarine

11 tablespoons prepared pancake mix

11 tablespoons all-purpose flour

$^1/_3$ cup evaporated skim milk

Topping:

1 teaspoon nutmeg

2 tablespoons brown sugar

1. Preheat oven to 400 degrees Fahrenheit.
2. Combine sugar, cinnamon, vanilla, cornstarch, pineapple juice, and peach nectar in a saucepan and cook over medium heat. Stir constantly until mixture thickens and bubbles.
3. Add sliced peaches and margarine to mixture.
4. Reduce heat and simmer for 5 to 10 minutes.
5. Pour hot peach mixture into lightly greased 4-inch-square glass dish.
6. In another bowl, combine pancake mix and flour. Stir in milk.
7. Quickly spoon this mixture over peach mixture.
8. Sprinkle on topping.
9. Bake for 25 to 30 minutes or until golden brown.
10. Cut into 6 squares.

SERVING SIZE: 1 SQUARE. MAKES 6 SERVINGS.

Calories   285   •   Fat   3 g   •   Saturated Fat   less than 1 g
Cholesterol   less than 1 mg   •   Sodium   240 mg

SUMMER BREEZES SMOOTHIE

1 cup plain nonfat yogurt

6 medium strawberries

1 cup crushed pineapple

1 medium banana

4 ice cubes

1. Place all ingredients in a blender and puree until smooth.
2. Serve in a frosty glass.

SERVING SIZE: 1 CUP. MAKES 2 SERVINGS.

Calories 176 • Fat 1 g • Saturated Fat less than 1 g
Cholesterol 2 mg • Sodium 89 mg

 # FRUITED VINEGAR

24 ounces rice vinegar or distilled vinegar

1 medium very ripe mango (or substitute 6 ounces of fresh fruit, such as pineapple, peaches, citrus, etc.)

1 small hot pepper, coarsely chopped

2 tablespoons ground allspice

1. Peel mango and cut into long 1-inch strips.
2. Combine mango and all other ingredients in an airtight jar.
3. Let sit for 1 to 2 weeks before using.
4. Spoon over vegetables or pasta salads.

SERVING SIZE: 1 TABLESPOON. MAKES 24 SERVINGS.

Calories 10 • Fat 0 • Saturated Fat 0
Cholesterol 0 • Sodium less than 1 mg

Appendix 4

HealthQuest Planners

HEALTHQUEST MENU COMPARISON WORKSHEET

	OLD MENU		NEW MENU	
Breakfast	Item	Calories	Item	Calories
	Total breakfast calories		Total breakfast calories	
Lunch				
	Total lunch calories		Total lunch calories	
Dinner				
	Total dinner calories		Total dinner calories	
Snack				
	Total snack calories		Total snack calories	
	TOTAL DAILY CALORIES		**TOTAL DAILY CALORIES**	

TOTAL CALORIES "OLD" MENU
-TOTAL CALORIES "NEW" MENU
=TOTAL CALORIES SAVED TODAY

HEALTHQUEST WEEKLY MENU PLANNER

Month _____
Week _____

Weight on Monday (lbs.) _____
Weight on Sunday (lbs.) _____

Day	Monday		Tuesday		Wednesday		Thursday		Friday		Saturday		Sunday	
	Food Item	Calories	Food Item	Calories	Food Item	Calories	Food Item	Calories	Food Item	Calories	Food Item	Calories	Food Item	Calories
Breakfast														
Total calories														
Lunch														
Total calories														
Dinner														
Total calories														
Snack														
Total calories														
DAILY TOTAL														
WEEKLY TOTAL														

HEALTHQUEST WEEKLY EXERCISE PLANNER

Month _____
Week _____

Weight on Monday (lbs.) _____
Weight on Sunday (lbs.) _____

Day	Monday	Tuesday	Wednesday	Thursday	Friday	Saturday	Sunday
Type of Exercise (list all)							
Stretches							
Cardiovascular/ Aerobic							
Strength Training Include exercise, amount of weight, number of reps, and number of sets							

Index

Index